MEDITATION, CONSCIOUSNESS, MIND:

The Habits That Will Change Your World

Table of Contents

Introduction

Chapter One: Subconscious Mind and Early Imprints

Chapter Two: Different Ways to Reprogram the Subconscious

Chapter Three: Meditation and Reprogramming the Subconscious

Chapter Four: Unlocking the Power of Dreams and Writing Consciousness

Chapter Five: Meditation and Lucid Dreaming

Chapter Six: Mindfulness and Mindful Meditation

Chapter Seven: Guided Visualization

Chapter Eight: Transforming Negative Thoughts Through Meditation

Conclusion

Introduction

A majority of our life is spent living in three states of consciousness – awake, dreaming and asleep. These states are represented by our conscious mind, subconscious mind and unconscious mind or the three levels of consciousness. In the 'awake' state of consciousness we are able to experience everything around us through the power of our five sense organs. Again, during the 'awake' state we engage in a number of activities. The opposite of this is the 'asleep' state of consciousness, where we are unaware of what is happening around us. In between these two states we are neither awake not asleep but dreaming or partially conscious/aware of what is happening around us.

The concept of consciousness still baffles human beings. There isn't a definite or conclusive explanation for it yet. However, what is clear is we can raise our own consciousness levels to fill the gap between the conscious and subconscious or unconscious mind to live a life of our dreams.

One of the best ways to work on your consciousness is to meditate. Meditation works at several levels. It increases your awareness, deepens your thought levels, enhances sensory perception and boosts your ability to process stimuli. There are plenty of other physical, mental, psychological and spiritual benefits of meditation. However, in this book we aim to understand the power of meditation in reprogramming your subconscious mind and helping you live the life you truly desire through positive thinking and living.

Again, it is challenging to explain the phenomenon of the subconscious. Though psychoanalysts have tried to nail a precise definition for the subconscious, it can only be described with ambiguity. In a way, our conscious and subconscious are intertwined.

The conscious mind is being utilized when you are awake to work, communicate with people, make decisions and perform other day-to-day activities. While the conscious mind is only the outer surface of our thought process, it is the subconscious mind that is filing away the main information, which is embedded in it almost forever. It is humanly impossible for us to try and absorb everything at a conscious level. Our minds would be overloaded.

Think of it this way. Throughout the day as we interact with people and perform our tasks, the subconscious mind is collecting, sorting and storing information for future.

Sometimes you are searching for an important thing all over the place but can't find it. You give up hope of finding it. However, suddenly on an impulse, you look for it in a place where you wouldn't usually keep it. And bingo, there it is! How did you know it was where you found it? The knowledge of where it was kept had been in your subconscious mind all along. However, only when it communicated with your conscious mind did you know where to find it.

Ever wondered what a "hunch" a "gut feeling" or "intuition" is? Often, it is nothing but a signal or communication from the subconscious mind to the conscious mind. Why are you asked to "sleep on your problems?" Simply because when we are asleep, our subconscious mind is most active.

When your subconscious' activity is at its peak, you can get some of the best insights and solutions to your problems simply because it holds information that is not accessible to our conscious mind. Some of our best solutions and "eureka" moments happen when we are asleep.

Has it happened several times that you've gone to bed thinking deeply about a problem with no solution in sight and suddenly you wake up with a solution and ask yourself why you hadn't thought of this before? It is your subconscious communicating with the conscious.

When you learn to reprogram your subconscious mind through meditation and positive thinking, you unlock or unleash the treasures or potential that have been held inside it for long. You can also use the power of meditation to restructure the imprints created in your subconscious mind during early years of your life.

Whether your goal is to lose weight, stop smoking, overcome addictions, get rid of a phobia, develop greater confidence or anything similar –you can use the power of meditation and positive thinking to manifest positive life goals.

Meditation is one of the best ways to unlock the power of the subconscious and deepen the connection between the conscious and subconscious. The deep sense of relaxation brought about by meditation facilitates filtering out distracting thoughts and allows you to concentrate only on the subconscious. When you allow a fresh lease of positive thoughts into the subconscious mind, negative information is replaced by more constructive thoughts and ideas. The mind is relaxed and receptive, open to assimilate positive information to replace negative imprints that have been accumulated over a period of time.

It won't be achieved overnight. However, with consistent and disciplined practice, you will be able to successfully reprogram the subconscious to hold thoughts, ideas, and information that hold a positive purpose in your life. You are slowly able to break the control of negative thoughts over your actions and let positive thoughts rule.

Research has proven that meditation possesses the ability to alter our brain waves. This increases the accessibility of your subconscious mind, letting you reprogram it to meet your goals.

Take a bunch of successful people from different fields and carefully notice what they have in common with each other. One of the things that will stand out is their thoughts or beliefs. They have successfully empowered themselves with virtues such as will-power, self-control, persistence and discipline.

There is an inner drive that pushes them to accomplish their goals. Our subconscious mind is the potent inner drive that helps unlock our true potential. There are plenty of people who are equally if not more talented that these successful people. However, not everyone enjoys their level of success, why? Simply because successful people have mastered of unlocking their true potential through the power of their thoughts or mind!

Meditation is the key to unlocking the power of your subconscious mind and using it to fulfill your dreams.

Chapter One: Subconscious Mind and Early Imprints

"Whatever we plant in our subconscious mind and nourish with repetition and emotion will one day become a reality."
– Earl Nightingale

Subconscious Mind Decoded

The subconscious mind is a state of dim or partial awareness, mainly comprising our dreams. It is a reservoir of experiences, beliefs and impressions left on our mind over the years. While our experiences leave behind impressions, the impressions in turn create or reinforce tendencies.

Every thought or every experience of gain and loss lives in our subconscious mind and creates a pattern of thoughts and actions. It impacts us at levels beyond our understanding. Unlike our conscious mind, the subconscious mind is not tamed by strict forces of the conscious mind. It is closely connected to a flow of ideas laced with intuition. However, what makes the ideas beliefs held in the subconscious challenging to change is the fact that they are not directed by logic but subjectivity. Often, when we dream and operate on the subconscious level, it may not be in tandem with the real world.

Again, the ideas, beliefs and experiences of the subconscious can easily occupy the conscious mind and trick the person into believing that they are being guided by intuition or a higher plane. What we believe to be intuition or higher guidance is in fact influenced by unfulfilled desires, past experiences and overall impressions. Since the subconscious is closer to the super conscious (true intuition) the two levels of consciousness represent an awareness flow that is without logical obstacles.

Our subconscious mind is highly receptive to intuitions that are passed through the superconscious. Sometimes, we make disastrous decisions believing that we are responding to an intuition or higher guidance, when in fact we are merely responding to a preconditioned subconscious.

Subconscious Mind and Early Childhood Experiences

We all like to believe that we are completely in control of our thoughts and actions. You've been slightly surprised to know that you have limited control over what drives your behavior. It may seem impossible to believe at first, however, let me explain this further. Before taking any action or making a decision, we are utilizing our conscious mind. Not all your innumerable actions throughout the day are guided by the conscious mind. A major part of them are also driven by the subconscious. Actions that are driven by the subconscious are not within the scope of your control.

A majority of our beliefs are formed during our early childhood years. Only 10 percent of our mind is represented by the conscious mind. The subconscious represents a staggering 90 percent of your mind. Most of your habits, involuntary responses and beliefs are stored in the subconscious. Think of where your fight or flight response originates.

There is a gap between the conscious mind and subconscious mind, which is termed as the critical mind. It is partly conscious and partly subconscious. It is a sort of filter that is in place to bring a sense of connection between the two levels of consciousness and protect us. The critical mind determines what enters the realm of the subconscious and what doesn't.

Children below the age of eight don't have actively developed left or right brains, which also means that during these formative years their subconscious mind is the most active. This allows it to be programmed naturally through events and experiences, which become firmly imprinted in mind even during later years of our life. When our conscious mind is not yet developed, the power of the subconscious is at its peak. It is during this phase that a majority of our self-limiting beliefs get entrenched in mind. This is why we are gravely impacted by the seemingly innocuous yet gravely hurtful words of an exhausted parent or educators who don't show much patience.

Our critical mind begins to develop around the age of eight, which means whatever children absorb through their senses (seeing, feeling, hearing, etc.) before that directly makes its way into their subconscious mind minus the critical thinking or analysis. Unlike the conscious mind, our subconscious mind is always awake. This allows it to collect a staggering amount of data.

This is exactly why the subconscious mind is most programmable during early childhood years when our brains believe whatever is fed into it, bereft as we are of the powers of analytical thinking and the conscious mind. Your brain is only recording data per se and registering everything that is fed into it as true.

Notice how children often grow up with the same beliefs as their parents because they communicated the most with their parents when their mind was most malleable and unable to distinguish between facts and opinions through critical analysis. If you are scared of heights or believe money doesn't really come easily or true love doesn't exist, chances are your children are also most likely to grow up with similar beliefs.

Willingly or unwittingly, you have instilled or imprinted these ideas into their subconscious when it was most receptive. Until the age of eight, the human brain frequency is ruled by Theta waves, thus holding us in a hypnagogic trance-like state where we absorb everything that goes into our mind as the truth, which seldom changes during later years of our life. This trance-like state that children below eight operate in allows all the information and experiences to pass directly into the realm of the subconscious. The conscious mind is bypassed with the brain simply downloading information without analyzing if the information is positive or negative and valuable or useless.

A majority of our beliefs are created during early formative years through what we see, experience and hear. We don't question our experiences or programming. When an impatient teacher chides us for not being good at something, we believe it without questioning it, and eventually grow up believing we aren't good at something unless that thought is challenged by an equally powerful experience or programming.

Say, for instance, a child grows up in a house where he or she has been constantly told that they will never get a good job and salary if they don't bag good grades in school. The child grows with a subconscious belief that he or she is not fit for or not worthy of getting a good job because they didn't get high grades.

During hypnotism, a person's brain frequencies are brought down to the state (delta and theta) where your child is naturally in during the initial seven to eight years of their life. This means the child is on a naturally hypnotic brain frequency, where their brain is assimilating all knowledge, feelings, and perceptions indiscriminately. Scary as it sounds, your child is being programmed for their adult life during this critical development phase. This subconscious programming development phase runs 95 percent of your life as an adult.

The subconscious mind neither has logic nor humor, which means even seemingly innocuous words such as "are you mad?" or "get lost" are absorbed by the subconscious mind in their literal sense. Also, the subconscious mind is incapable of differentiating between the real and imagined. To it, everything that is fed into it is real. There is no imagination or imagined reality. This is exactly why self-help gurus advocate journaling your goals or visualizing your thoughts. It is because when you repeatedly vocalize, write or visualize your goals, you are sending powerful signals to the subconscious mind that they are real. The subconscious mind cannot distinguish between the real and the imagined, which simply means it believes everything that it absorbs as real. This helps it direct our actions in line with these goals.

Children catch helplessness or self-limiting behavior early in life because they are incapable of differentiating between opinions, suggestions, and facts. Suggestions and opinions often become embedded in their minds as facts.

They accept as truth what is told to them as an opinion, which becomes an intrinsic part of their belief or value system. The belief subsequently becomes deeply entrenched in the subconscious mind, often without us even knowing we hold these beliefs until they are tested. There is a direct link between how children feel and their behavior.

It is only between the ages of ten to twelve that the child begins to develop reasoning powers and logic. They become capable of making decisions and exercising willpower. While the left-brain hemisphere is associated with critical thinking, the right brain hemisphere is linked with creativity.

Younger kids are vulnerable to negative suggestions because they accept them with the same frequency as positive ones. Therefore, if a child's core belief system comprises fear, lack of self-esteem, rejection, inadequacy, lack of confidence, etc. in the subconscious mind, their decisions will invariably reflect these negative beliefs.

The good news is that these beliefs can be worked upon by meditation and positive thinking. Our brain can be replaced with more positive and constructive thoughts to eliminate negative thoughts held in it over a period of time. Through relaxation and mindfulness, we can move into different levels of consciousness to train the mind to think and therefore act in a specific, positive manner.

Chapter Two: Different Ways to Reprogram the Subconscious

"You must take personal responsibility. You cannot change the circumstances, the seasons, or the wind, but you can change yourself." – Jim Rohn

There are several proven techniques through which a person can reprogram their subconscious mind, which can eventually transform the way they think about life and themselves. This can make the process of goal manifestation or changing your life easier.

Without you even realizing it, a major chunk of your life is dictated by the subconscious mind. Don't agree? Read on.

Just visualize a waterfall with two different paths below it through which water can possibly flow.

If the water consistently flows to only through one particular path, the path starts expanding and deepening. It obstructs the chances of water flowing through the other path. Over a period of time, the other path is filled with dirt and sand, while the path through which water regularly flows becomes the sole direction for the water to flow in. Eventually, the unused path may dry up and disappear.

Similarly, our mind forms associations and connections about all ideas we experience. There are neural connections established in the brain through which our behavior is determined.

We lend meaning to each association of experience we encounter. The entire process of offering specific meanings to experiences that are encountered by us in everyday life, our memory through various encounters, the formation of beliefs, our unique personality and more is a nothing but a group of associations that we've built over time.

Though the human brain has 100 billion neurons that have the capacity to form 100 trillion different neural associations, we utilize only a fraction of these. Our focus and thoughts are always traveling through limited pathways though there are several other potential pathways, which means we are not exploring the full power of our mind. If we keep reinforcing the same associations without restructuring them or forming new associations, we are not unlocking the true power of our mind.

Let us look at an example, think of an incident during your childhood when you were bitten by a dog. Since that day, the image of a dog has been associated with fear and pain. Your instant reaction based on this association (dog-fear) is to escape. So, each time you see a dog, you have the same reaction to run. You are not allowing your mind to create new associations. Now, just imagine initiating a change in this association by befriending the dog rather than running away.

On befriending the dog, you realize that it can indeed be a friendly creature, which allows you to form new associations.

Here are some secrets to unlock the potential of your subconscious mind.

1. Positive Affirmations

Using positive affirmations makes it easier for us to train the subconscious through the power of repetition. Affirmations are nothing but positive and personal statements repeated in the present tense several times throughout the day. They are meant to challenge a pre-held and limiting negative self-belief. For instance, let's assume you are low on confidence and socially awkward while meeting new people. With affirmations, you will seek to challenge the notion by saying something like, "I am a confident person who attracts lots of friends and social acquaintances."

The act of repetition a powerful, positive statement is done with the intention of allowing this positive thought to override the negative self-belief held within the mind. I know several people who like to repeat affirmations while meditating to make its impact even more effectual.

The thing about our subconscious mind is that it is unable to differentiate between the real and imaginary. When you talk about something as if you already have it, the mind is quickly led into believing that it is nothing but the truth. When you say, "you are a confident person who attracts lots of friends and social acquaintances," you are simply tricking your subconscious mind into believing what you want to create as already true.

Once it believes you are indeed a confident person, it directs your actions precisely in line with this belief. This makes your subconscious-directed actions and behavior even more confident, self-assured and open to socializing. It won't come immediately, but there will be a gradual shift in the way you start perceiving and approaching things around you.

There are new pathways created within the subconscious through repetition, which makes manifesting your goal even easier. These new pathways bring about a gradual shift in your attitude, thus allowing your actions to be driven by the mind in a more positive direction.

When you say, "I choose happiness, gratitude and peace at all times" you are shifting the mindset from anger, disappointment and sadness. Always keep affirmations in the present tense, while also making them detailed and personal.

Avoid using negative words while saying your affirmations. For example, instead of saying, "I do not want to be sad today" say, "I am happy today" or "I choose to be happy today."

Keep the words simple and affirmations pithy. You don't have to use big, fancy words. Instead, use signals that are easily understood by the subconscious mind. Keep your words/phrases small, relevant and powerful. This will bring about a shift in your thought process.

Affirmations can be stuck on notes, which can be prominently placed around your home and office. Think about the wall opposite your bed, which is the first thing you spot each morning, or your bathroom mirror. How about your dressing table, cupboard, refrigerator and work desk? These will act as gentle, inspiring and positive reminders of who you desire to be. Become as creative as you want while creating your affirmations while retaining their essence and meaning.

The more these affirmations are repeated, the more effectively they will be integrated into your subconscious realm, thus making your thought process stronger and more positive. From operating with a "lack of" perception, you will start operating with an "abundance" perception. Instead of believing you are not a confident and socially savvy person, your subconscious will accept that you are a confident and socially savvy person, thus leading your actions in line with this positive thought.

Create a positive mantra that you can chant during meditation. When anxiety and stress increase, mantra can calm the mind in a positive manner. Consistently using a mantra will allow you to mitigate negative thoughts and eliminating self-limiting beliefs. Create a healing mantra that challenges your judgmental or self-limiting beliefs.

2. Hypnosis

Hypnosis is a form of therapy that is used to bring about a change in the thought pattern of the subconscious mind by drawing it into a state of extreme relaxation, where it is ready to absorb everything that is fed into it. This is the stage when the conscious mind is able to let go of its hold, and the subconscious takes over. The latter can be effortlessly reprogrammed into absorbing new beliefs, thoughts, ideas and more during the process of hypnosis.

3. Visualization

Visualization is another powerful technique for manifesting your goals or bringing the desired changes in your life. It is the process through which you create precise, detailed and vivid mental visuals to accomplish the intended outcome.

The idea is to pass these images into the realm of the subconscious mind when it is in a highly receptive state.

Visualization or guided visual meditation allows the mind to form mental visuals of what it seeks. These purposeful and meaningful mental images subsequently lead the subconscious mind into absorbing it as reality. Our actions, attitude, and behavior are then channelized by the mind towards accomplishing these goals. Notice the difference in your self-esteem when you start using affirmations to accomplish any goal.

4. Meditation

Meditation techniques allow you to calm and reprogram the mind when it is in a more receptive state. There are several meditation techniques that allow you to access different levels of consciousness using visualization, mindfulness, imagination, focus and more. If you want the subconscious mind to submit into a specific way of thinking or behaving, meditation can help you accomplish it.

The power to create what you desire lies in your subconscious mind. You only need to unlock the potential of the mind through various meditation and other positive thinking techniques.

Determine what exactly you want in life. Make short and precise statements about it. For instance, "I am the owner of xyz business in 2018." Keep repeating this statement to yourself all the time. Write it in a place where you are likely to see it, and it gets firmly entrenched in your subconscious mind.

Keep looking at your goal statements throughout the day and keep repeating them. Meditate on these goals. Visualize yourself as already having fulfilled these goals. Continue these exercises for at least 3 weeks-4 weeks, and you'll begin to observe a shift in the way you perceive your goals and your ability to fulfill these goals. You'll develop a renewed sense of hopefulness and positivity. There will be a clear shift in your attitude, actions, and behavior.

5. Journaling

Journaling is another fantastic way to tap into the inexhaustive reserves of the subconscious mind. By giving form to your goals and writing them in a flowing stream of consciousness, you are simply sending powerful signals to your subconscious mind.

When writing about our deepest desires or goals, we are again leading the subconscious mind along with other levels of consciousness to think of these goals as real and not imagined. Through the act of writing something or giving something a tangible form, you allow the subconscious mind to internalize your goals.

Resist the urge to edit or structure your thoughts and allow them to flow in a more unrestrained manner. Your writing should be personal to reflect your thoughts and feelings. Let the writing flow in a steady stream of consciousness. The physical act of writing and our subconscious mind is closely connected. When you give a physical form to your thoughts or ideas, it has a higher chance of being absorbed by the subconscious mind.

Like we already know by now, the subconscious mind is unable to differentiate between the real and imagined. What makes its way into the subconscious is always deemed as real by it. When you start writing about a clear goal or dream, the mind doesn't see it as something you wish to accomplish but as something that is already a part of your life. Thus, it drives your actions or behavior to match these goals, which helps you achieve them. You are doing nothing but unlocking the power of your subconscious mind in fulfilling these goals.

You can either go with a single journal or keep multiple journals with different themes. For instance, I know people who have a gratitude journal, goal journal, dream journal (to note down the dreams you experience throughout the time you are asleep), affirmations journal and more.

One of the best ways to bring about a change in the feelings held within your consciousness is to keep a gratitude journal.

Write ten things that you feel blessed to have in your life at the end of each day (before going to bed when your subconscious is at its peak).

Try to come up with a different set of blessings to be grateful for every day. Be thankful for everything from the eyes that allow you to view the beautiful world around you to the legs that carry you around to the shelter above your head to the internet that allows you to connect with the world. You'll be surprised at how much you have to be thankful for. The simple act of being thankful for your gifts allows your subconscious to draw even greater blessings. You are tapping into the subconscious and allowing it to receive powerful signals. This ultimately molds your thoughts and actions.

Look around you carefully even when you believe you don't have much to be grateful for. This will help you come up with plenty of blessings and lead your mind into a more positive, hopeful and constructive frame of mind, which will allow it to manifest or create more blessings. Your mind becomes receptive to even more blessings, thus helping you harness the potential of positive thinking. The best time to write a gratitude journal is just before going to bed when the subconscious mind is at its peak.

Similarly, if you are recording your dreams to understand what is held within the subconscious mind, note your dreams as soon as you wake up in the morning. Once you are fully awake and the conscious mind takes over, it becomes challenging to recall the signals or messages from the subconscious.

Chapter Three: Meditation and Reprogramming the Subconscious

"Your attitude not your aptitude determines your altitude."
– Anonymous

Meditation is one of the most powerful tools for activating the potential of the subconscious mind, reprogramming our thoughts or increasing the power of our subconscious. Meditation is known to possess multiple physical, mental and psychological benefits as consistently concluded by researchers.

Through meditation, a practitioner can relieve stress, improve focus, increase creativity/productivity, reignite their cognitive thinking powers and much more. It helps us draw the things we want in life and fulfill our goals.

There are five fundamental brainwave categories in our brain, where each matches with our actions and thoughts. The main objective of meditation is to slow the pace of our brain waves to create greater time duration between thoughts. This gives us the power to pick the thoughts that we want to nurture, and actions we desire to take guided by these thoughts. When there are too many thoughts occupying our mind with a shorter gap, our thoughts become involuntary. We have little control over what to invest our thought energy in, and what actions to perform as a result of those thoughts.

Rules for Reprogramming the Subconscious Mind

1. Be clear about what you desire

Reprogramming your subconscious mind begins with a clear understanding of what you want to change or the goals you want to accomplish. For example, let us assume you are raised with the belief that you aren't good enough for anything or that you are worthy of rejection, and therefore are low on confidence. You recognize that fact that you lack confidence, which you want to change. The belief that you are unworthy of accomplishing anything substantial in life has been deeply ingrained in you, but you want to challenge that belief or bring about a change in your thought process.

To reprogram your subconscious mind through meditation and other techniques, it is important to identify what exactly you want. What are the areas that you need to work on? What are the goals you desire to accomplish?

Ideally, focus on a single goal at a time. If you try to fulfill too many scattered goals, you'll stop being goal-oriented. For example, if you are looking for a soulmate, don't cloud that goal with weight loss goals, attracting more money, overcoming stress, etc. Focus only on your quest for a perfect soulmate.

2. Identify subconscious patterns that block you

Once you have identified a clear goal, identify subconscious patterns that block you from having a conversation with yourself. Find subconscious patterns and challenges that define the big picture.

For example, if you are looking for a perfect soulmate or partner, you need to have an objective and honest conversation with yourself about what is holding you back from finding the right person. Get rid of all the masks and think about everything that is stopping you from meeting this person. Do you come across as too emotionally dependent which makes prospective partners run in another direction? Do you suffer from low self-confidence or self-esteem, which is unappealing to potential mates?

Identify your subconscious blockages to help eliminate them gradually. For example, if your parents held high expectations from you all the time and never seemed to be happy with what you accomplished, you may grow up with a low sense of self-worth. This low sense of self-worth may be preventing you from attracting the right partners because you are constantly seeking acceptance.

When you recognize that these are early childhood subconscious beliefs you are operating with, you know what you are up against. These subconscious mental blockages that hold you back are easier to eliminate once you identify them.

3. Subconscious shift methods are most effective before going to sleep

One of the best times to bring about a change or shift in your subconscious is to use techniques for reprogramming the subconscious just before going to bed or first thing in the morning. This is the time when your subconscious is at its peak. Around 15-20 minutes before going to bed, the body and mind begin to relax. Our body's muscles ease up a bit, and the heartbeat slows down. The entire body slips into a state of relaxation. The brain subsequently generates alpha waves.

EEG research reveals that during this 15-20-minute gap between being awake and falling asleep, the brain waves reduce to 7-14 alpha waves per second. This is the time when the subconscious mind is most receptive to messages.

This is precisely why self-help and goal manifestation gurus advocate practicing visualizations, journaling, and affirmations right before going to bed. Since the passage of the subconscious is most open and receptive to assimilating ideas while going to bed and even while we are asleep, it is able to absorb the message more effectively.

Meditation and Breathing

Meditation is not challenging to begin with. It can be as simple as being more mindful of your everyday actions or focusing on your breath. Unlike what people may have you believe, it isn't spiritual mumbo-jumbo or a full-fledged ritual complete with incense sticks, candles, and figurines. Just pick a place where you can sit peacefully and comfortably, without much disturbance. Relax your body and keep an erect posture. Keep your hands relaxed on the lap and shut your eyes.

You simply follow your breath and notice your breathing pattern in a silent, relaxed and mindful manner. Practice breathing in and breathing out in a rhythm directed by the mind! Each time you find the mind the wandering or getting distracted, gently draw it back to the breath. When the breathing becomes slow, your mind becomes calmer.

Positive Thinking Through Meditation

When a kid walks on sand, he/she creates tiny footprints or impressions on the sand. Similarly, when an adult walks the same path, the kid's footprints are automatically erased and replaced with the adult's footprints. The smaller footprint trail is erased, while the larger one stays. Think of all the negative thinking you've accumulated in different levels of consciousness as negative footprints.

Meditation is designed to take an individual to the core of his being or the source of his existence. The core of our being is filled with positivity, joy, and creativity. If you are able to tap into this source to bring about a positive change in your life, meditation is one of the more effective techniques to accomplish it.

What you are attempting to do is to erase tinier footprints with larger footprints that are filled with greater positivity. Regularly accessing the core of your being helps you tap into the subconscious mind to bring about a series of positive changes in your life.

If you want to draw the right things in your life like a magnet, your thoughts, beliefs, perceptions, and expectations should be in line with receiving these positives.

If your thoughts are fundamentally overcome by fear, stress, worry, anxiety, and depression, you will draw even more experiences that reinforce these negative thoughts. The secret is to allow the power of positive thinking to operate in your favor. Meditation attempts to change and restructure your thoughts from the subconscious layers.

Once the layers of stress, depression, anxiety and fear free your mind, the subconscious mind is de-clogged. The layers of negative thinking are replaced by more clarity in thoughts and actions. Thus, a positive attitude and positive techniques such as meditation allow you to manifest everything you want in life.

Meditation is an exercise for the mind. Just like physical activities award you greater physical strength and stamina, meditation increases the mind's neurostimulation and leads the nervous system to function at its optimal capacity.

A meditation practitioner's nervous system is altered and restructured to access new levels. A regular and disciplined meditation practice creates new neural pathways, thus leading to a transformation in your thought and behavior. Communication between your left and right hemisphere increases, thus facilitating more integrated brain functioning.

Innumerable studies conducted in the EEG (electroencephalograph) domain reveal that some of the world's most successful people have their brain's two hemispheres working in tandem with each other. Meditation allows our left and right brain to work in unison, a term referred to as "brain synchronization." There are several beneficial changes including enhanced blood flow and brain chemistry.

Chapter Four: Unlocking the Power of Dreams and Writing Consciousness

The first step towards bringing about a change in your subconscious mind is to understand what's held inside it. When you are able to identify the underlying thoughts, feelings, beliefs and attitudes that are locked within the multiple layers of consciousness, it is easier to bring about a shift in them through meditation. The trickiest part of our subconscious mind is that it doesn't communicate with our senses like the conscious mind. You have to tune in to its deepest feelings by relaxing and allow your thoughts to flow in a stream of consciousness, without any obstacles.

This can be achieved through writing in a flow of consciousness and noting your dreams. Here are two powerful ways that can be combined with meditation to bridge the gap between multiple layers of consciousness.

1. Stream of writing consciousness

Keep a paper and pen ready and set a timer for 5-10 minutes. Keep away all distractions. Put your phone on silent mode. Do not use a gadget for writing your thoughts.

Sit in a comfortable posture and practice deep breathing for a few minutes before you begin writing. Center your focus on the breath. Begin the timer and start writing immediately. Don't have any pre-set agenda for what you are going to write. Stream of consciousness thoughts should flow naturally without any pre-determined agenda. Let the thoughts pour naturally and move from one into another without thinking too much about it.

As thoughts occupy your mind, put them on paper. Don't edit them or think about what to write and omit. However mundane, odd or pointless the thoughts feel, write them. These are often thoughts that originate from the subconscious and point to fundamental feelings held in the mind. Avoid the tendency to judge, rationalize or overanalyze these thoughts as they are often outside the scope of our logical mind. Continue writing these thoughts as they occur and stop only once the timer buzzes.

Once you are done writing or recording your stream of consciousness thoughts, read everything you've penned. Reflect on your choice of words. Is there a specific pattern in the words or phrases you use? For example, do you constantly find yourself writing words such "I am not good enough" or "I do not feel worthy enough" or "I don't think I deserve it" in the writing? Does it point to low self-esteem or self-acceptance?

Similarly, is there a theme or pattern in your thoughts? For instance, "this happened to me" or "this is why I wasn't able to do this" or "they did this to me." Are you always blaming other people and circumstances for everything that happens to you? Look for an overriding pattern in your thoughts and words.

Do several such writing sessions. While reading your current session, go back to previous sessions and note if there is a match or underlying theme between previous writings and the current session.

Note a few potential subconscious ideas you hold. Trace the progress or evolution of your thoughts once you begin meditating and practicing positive thinking using strategies described in other chapters. Note if your subconscious thoughts have transformed over a period of time owing to the different meditation exercises.

Practice Dream Analysis

Recording your dreams is another powerful way to tap into multiple layers of consciousness to understand what exactly is held within them. Before going to bed, keep a pen and dream journal adjacent to your bed.

When you awake in the morning or frequently throughout the night, record your dreams exactly as they occurred however ridiculous they appear to you. Mention all the details vividly. The act of noting your dreams should be done first thing in the morning because the impressions of these dreams will slowly get fainter as the day progresses and your conscious mind takes over. Mention every detail that you can think of vividly. Do not miss anything, however trivial, mundane and inconsequential it appears to you.

Is there a pattern in your dreams? Like not studying for an important exam or going for a job interview unprepared? This may reveal feelings of stress, anxiety or underperforming at important events. Observe the themes and underlying emotions behind your dreams. How do you feel after the dream? What is the deeper meaning behind the dream? When you are done recording your dreams over a period of time, note any recurring concepts, themes, objects, and characters.

Our subconscious mind often reveals itself through your dreams. Therefore, recording and analyzing dreams allows you to access otherwise inaccessible areas of the subconscious.

Determine the significance and category of dreams. Not all dreams may be significant or reveal the underlying emotions of our subconscious mind. Dreams that involve senses such as sounds, physical actions, and smells may not point to feelings or thoughts locked within the subconscious. Dreams related to the subconscious are often bizarre and perplexing. Again, within significant dreams, there can be different categories. Determine which category of significance your dreams fall under.

Is it a precognitive dream that determines specific, accurate details about future events? This is what is termed as a premonition or insight about events that occur in future. Is your subconscious communicating with you about events that are about to unfold in the future? Is the dream meant to serve as a warning for future events? Is the dream a reinforcement of facts you are already aware of? Did the dream awaken you to a truth or inspire action? Did you fulfill a strong desire in the dream? Did you mend bridges with a person? Dreams that are more vivid and detailed are the ones that you need to watch out for.

Sometimes, the solution to your most pressing problems will come in the form of a dream. When you go to bed thinking persistently about a problem that your conscious is unable to find a solution for, the subconscious takes over when you are sleeping. This is exactly why most solutions to our pressing problems occur when we "sleep on it." When our conscious mind is asleep, the subconscious is at its peak. This is why insights that are beyond the scope of our conscious mind come easier to the subconscious mind.

Interpret or analyze your dreams. You don't have to be an ace psychologist to interpret your own dreams! It just needs some reading and understanding. Plenty of resources are available on the internet related to dream interpretation. Read your dream in its entirety rather than standalone parts. Recall as many details as you can about the dream, which will make the interpretation even more power-packed.

Not everything you read in a dream interpretation dictionary may be applicable in your own life. Relate the dream to your life, and the context of current events you are facing.

For example, let's say you see a dream about someone pushing you in deep water, where you don't know how to swim and struggle for survival. A dream dictionary may interpret this dream as an act of betrayal by someone close to you. However, if you have a job interview coming up and you feel the weight of other people's expectations on you, the dream may signify you don't feel prepared enough to handle other people's expectations, or you don't feel you are prepared for the job or interview. Therefore, it is important to identify a dream within the context of your life or current events unfolding within your life to make the interpretation more effectual.

Try to understand if there is a reason why a person, object or event occurred in your dream, and attempt to relate it to your life.

Once you get into the flow of analyzing your dreams, you'll begin to decode your subconscious and unconscious thoughts with even greater accuracy.

Chapter Five: Meditation and Lucid Dreaming

Lucid dreaming is an established scientific technique for gaining a deeper awareness of our dreams. This simply means that when you are dreaming, you are aware of the fact that that are you dreaming, and pretty much able to control the flow of your dreams. You can explore how you want the dream to go or control the outcome of your dreams.

When we are otherwise dreaming, we aren't generally aware of the fact that we are dreaming. There is a blurring line between dreams and reality in minds, with the two often overlapping. You are not in control of how your dreams pan out.

With lucid dreaming, you are completely aware of the fact that you are dreaming, and have the power to explore, imagine and control your dreams. Meeting a famous personality, becoming a more confident public speaker, getting a dream job, owning a house is all possible within the realm of lucid dreaming.

Lucid dreaming is possible because while you are asleep your mind remains awake and it is able to experience things. Normally, your brain simply shuts off, and you are unaware of what is happening inside it.

However, with sufficient training and practice, you can open the part of your mind that is responsible for being more aware of what is happening. When you are aware of where to steer your dreams, there is no limit to what you can imprint in the subconscious mind.

Lucid dreaming is a scientifically proven phenomenon that was first used by Tibetan monks, and later by several successful people around the world to unlock the power of their subconscious mind through dreams and meditation.

Though everyone could practice lucid dreaming, not all will because much like other abilities, it requires training, practice to develop the habit. Once you get into the habit of meditating and lucid dreaming, it can be fun and insightful. You'll uncover plenty of thoughts held in different layers of consciousness that you weren't aware of. Once you are aware of these thoughts and feelings that have been accumulated within the subconscious for long, it will be easier bring about a positive shift in them.

Through lucid dreaming, you are attempting to reprogram the mind into acting in a way it hasn't considered before due to pre-set notions. It will take some trial and effort on your part to master meditating on your dreams. The more you practice, the more effectively you'll be able to train your mind to think and act in ways that are beneficial to you. It can take anywhere from 10 to 30 nights to master lucid dreaming depending on every person's mind and thought process.

Here are some reasons why meditation facilitates the process of lucid or on-demand dreaming.

Lucid dreams are a highly complex phenomenon. In effect, you are trying to fill the gap between the conscious and subconscious mind. This unnatural merger of the free-thinking subconscious and the rational conscious can lead to a clash.

The conscious mind can be a huge saboteur of lucid dreaming owing to the fact that it entertains plenty of unwanted, negative and stray thoughts. Now, you have to make the conscious mind behave in a more controlled manner, so it doesn't disturb the lucid dreaming manner. How do you train the untamed conscious mind to behave?

Enter meditation. As the dream spins around and there is total chaos in the mind, meditation can help you gain a higher perspective, become more self-aware and control the direction of your thoughts. It helps you witness the unfolding of your dreams in more objective and emotionally detached manner. Meditation helps you accomplish a state where your mind is awake and active, even while the body is asleep to stay relaxed, calm and in control before, during and post a lucid dream.

Lucid Dreaming

One of the most important points to keep in mind when you practice lucid dreaming is to keep doing a reality check by questioning yourself. Are you dreaming? Are the dreams for real? Doing a real-time dream check will allow you to instill heightened attention from the conscious mind into the dream. Therefore, your conscious mind will establish a greater connection with the subconscious mind to increase your attention and awareness of the dream, thus creating a form of instant lucidity.

Meditation fills the gap between the sleeping and waking mind. You are injecting more awareness of your conscious mind into what is essentially an unconscious or subconscious process. Meditation essentially creates a bridge or link between multiple layers of consciousness, which can be used to restructure your mind in a more positive manner.

Mindfulness earned through meditation helps our conscious mind become aware of the fact that we are dreaming. In addition to this, the conscious mind learns to enjoy the process with lesser distractions and greater positivity.

Here are some tips and techniques to get you started with lucid dreaming meditation.

Start by relaxing the body and mind. When you are trying to achieve an "out of the body" feeling, relaxing your senses and mind is vital. It'll require plenty of willpower and practice, so prepare yourself physically and mentally for the experience.

We'll go through some meditation techniques that will help you enjoy a more relaxed sleep, and gather greater energy, which will increase your likelihood of being able to practice more effective lucid dreaming.

If you've seen *The Matrix,* in the beginning, Neo is offered a choice by Morpheus. The first alternative is a blue pill, letting Neo keep everything that he has built during the course of his life intact. Nothing he has built over a period of his life will change.

The second alternative is to take the red pill, which introduces Neo to the truth that any reality is purely a construction or creation of his mind, that exists on the basis of his beliefs, ideas, and thoughts.

Which of the two pills do you think is integral to the process to lucid dreaming? Yes, you got it right, the red pill!

We go through our daily lives in a more mechanical or clinical manner paying little attention to, or developing little awareness of what is happening around us. We often mindlessly accept whatever we are presented with exactly as it is. For example, you know that you cannot float in the air because of gravity or that you cannot penetrate walls.

The blue pill, on the surface, appears to be a better option. You can retain things exactly as they are. This is pretty much what everyone around you is doing. Attempting to keep their thoughts gained over a period of time intact. There is little self-awareness or connection with your mind. This lack of awareness or unchanging thoughts makes lucid dreaming challenging.

The red pill, on the other hand, doesn't limit your thoughts or keep them unchanged. It helps you construct your reality through thoughts, which is the purpose of lucid dreaming. In a sense, you are not leaving previous thoughts unchallenged but creating a new reality for yourself through the power of thoughts. These thoughts will eventually determine the course of your actions.

Through the red pill, we aren't limiting ourselves to the information held in our conscious mind or what "we know." We are attempting to unleash the power of information that has been inaccessible to us yet contains the power to transform our lives if challenged.

Use a powerful visualization technique to increase your ability to create and control dream sequences that restructure the thoughts in your subconscious mind.

Visualization One

Begin by sitting or lying down in a comfortable position. Shut your eyes, loosen up your body and allow the muscles to relax.

Now slowly visualize yourself walking on a pristine and beautiful island. Imagine the gorgeous island as vividly as you can by involving your senses. What are the sights and sounds you experience? How do you feel when you walk through the island? What are the thoughts that occupy your mind? Visualize walking through the balmy, shallow and blue waters of the island.

Move into the warm, golden sand. Notice how it feels against your feet. Visualize the feeling of the sun's rays touching your body. Imagine that a sudden warm wave splashes water on your face. Each person will visualize the same scenario in different ways depending on their thoughts, ideas, perceptions, and feelings. Let your imagination run free. Try to explore the island using your own ideas and interpretations. Add your own details. I also recommend using guided meditation music throughout the session.

As you keep exploring and discovering the island, focus on this one thought, "I am actually dreaming, and I am completely aware of the fact that I am dreaming." This makes the process of meditation, visualization and lucid dreaming more effective.

Keep going with the visualization for 10-15 minutes (set a timer). Once the session ends, write your experience in detail in a dream journal. Do this exercise just before you sleeping to heighten your sense of awareness.

Come up with visual dream scenes of your choice and explore them as you wish to create an outcome you desire. Form visualizations based on the lucid dreams you wish to have.

For instance, if you want to have a lucid dream about performing exceptionally well in a job interview, create visualizations around the scene with an outcome of your choice. This will increase the likelihood of seeing lucid dreams that unfold with a more positive outcome.

Lucid dreaming is more effective when your mind is relaxed, open and in a semi-consciousness state. You should be able to access realms of the subconscious and unconscious to facilitate the practice of lucid dreaming.

Visualization Two

Let us take another guided meditation exercise that helps you focus and increases self-awareness while increasing the power of different consciousness layers.

Imagine walking through a lush, green and beautiful garden that looks like paradise. It is natural, untamed and never-ending! There are no boundaries from where it begins and ends, it is just infinite. Imagine the pure, clean air in the pristine garden filling up your lungs. Observe the beauty and serenity around you.

The idea is to use the power of positive images and settings to free negative and stressful thoughts held in the mind. Tune in intently and purposefully to the silence that occupies the space. Hear trees hustling and swooshing in a peaceful backdrop. Listen to the sound of birds chirping in the background. Notice the haunting sound of raindrops falling on the ground and surface of the trees in a rhythm.

Feel the soft texture of grass below your bare feet. Touch the flowers and leaves. Feel the cool, soft and fresh air moving around you. Take time to savor each moment and experience as it is happening. Explore the serene garden for as long as you like. Witness walking on different paths of the garden! Go deeper and deeper into the garden path as you attempt to access different levels of consciousness.

There is a strong link between meditation and lucid dreaming. Both these techniques are known to involve states of awareness that are higher than the conscious mind. They help increase focus, self-awareness, and reflection. You are able to recall dreams more effectively and enhance your visualization skills to tap into the subconscious mind.

Continue walking and focus on the scenery that keeps changing all the time. Explore a gentle slope within the garden. Imagine this slope as different layers consciousness that allows you to go deeper and deeper into the realm of consciousness. Imagine penetrating through different layers of your mind or consciousness as you go down the slope.

It takes around 15 minutes-20 minutes for the body to assume a trance-like state, with minimal awareness of the physical body. Stay in the trance-like state for as long as you wish since there really is no limit to the areas of the mind you can access in this relaxed, trance state.

Finally, when you feel ready to get back to the real world, gently get yourself up from the trance state by counting from ten to one. Take deep breaths as you slowly count backward and rouse yourself from the trance. Give yourself some time to get accustomed to the real, while slowly opening your eyes. Again, the idea of this exercise is to eliminate distractions and heighten self-awareness, which is vital for lucid dreams. Form and explore your own inner worlds. Keep it different and creative each time, as long it facilitates a sense of calmness, relaxation, positivity and detailed mental imagery.

Chapter Six: Mindfulness and Mindful Meditation

"The best way to capture moments is to pay attention. This is how we cultivate mindfulness." – Jon Kabat-Zinn

Mindful meditation will allow you to focus on the power of your subconscious mind. Mindfulness is a purposeful and nonjudgmental awareness of the present moment. It is about completely absorbing the present by focusing on it in with intention and objectivity. Being mindful means being completely aware of the present, without dwelling on thoughts of the past and future! It can be practiced not just in meditation but everything from mindful walking to mindful eating to mindful driving.

Here's how to practice mindfulness to unleash the power of your subconscious mind.

Preparing to Meditate

Begin by determining the duration of your meditation. When you are starting, do not meditate for more than 5-10 minutes. Wear comfortable clothes and sit in a relaxed posture. Pick a location that is distraction and clutter-free. A serene, relaxed and inspiring location allows you to focus. Stretch before beginning the session and assume a comfortable seating posture on a chair or floor. Use cushions for support. Release tension from your body and relax your back and shoulders.

Establish Posture

Find a comfortable seating and sit straight on a chair with feet planted on the ground or sit cross-legged on the floor atop a pillow. Position your upper arms parallel to the two body sides. Keep the elbows slightly bent, while the hands should be on your knees. The chin should be little lowered to fix your gaze on the floor. Settle into a comfortable posture for gaining greater awareness of the body.

Focus on your Breathing

Shut your eyes and start following your breath. Focus on the process of inhaling and exhaling. Relax, and let the mind wander. Let the thoughts flow from the subconscious mind into the realm of the conscious. When the mind wanders, gently bring draw it back to the present.

Fleetingly note these thoughts but avoid judging them. Let these thoughts complete their course and pass. Once you realize the mind is wandering, gently focus your attention back on the breath. Your mind will keep wandering throughout the session as thoughts pass from the subconscious into the conscious. Be mindful of these thoughts and draw the mind back to your breath. Repeat this several times during the session.

Benefits of Mindfulness for the Subconscious

What impact does mindfulness have on the subconscious? If you come across thoughts held in the subconscious mind every day, does it automatically mean you are being more mindful?

1. Mindfulness impacts your learning abilities and memory. Research studies also found a greater density of grey matter in the brain's hippocampus that is known to be an important brain region for compassion, introspection and self-awareness.

2. Mindfulness is known to increase the brain's intuitive powers to award you flashes based on what is held within the subconscious mind. The intuitive flashes originate instincts habits and opinions. Therefore, mindfulness allows you to

establish a more effective connection with higher levels of consciousness. So, in effect, tuning in to these higher levels of consciousness or intuition may lead you in the right direction.

3. Mindfulness enhances your creative abilities since our subconscious mind holds limitless creativity. It also has huge reserves of potentially powerful information and plenty of untapped potentials.

4. Sometimes we don't have a clear understanding of our phobias and fears. Mindfulness can help you access deeper regions of the mind to unlock the reality of these fears. For example, a person may be suspicious of everyone around him and have a deep fear when it comes to trusting people.

These deep-seated fears are often planted in the subconscious through early childhood experiences. With a more enhanced connection with the subconscious, you can step back and observe these feelings in a more objective manner to understand its root cause.

5. Mindfulness successfully brings about a greater clarity of thoughts. You can dig deep into multiple layers of consciousness and be more mindful of your words, thoughts, and actions.

Practicing Mindfulness in Daily Life

Mindfulness makes it easier for you connect with deeper states of consciousness by increasing self-awareness, becoming more purposeful and observing the present in a nonjudgmental manner. When you practice mindfulness in everyday life, you stop functioning on autopilot and are therefore more aware of the thoughts and feelings held inside the subconscious mind.

Mindfulness is not just a meditation technique but a way of life that allows you to control the way you perceive the world. You learn to exist in the present moment and increase your awareness of the present. There is greater control over things you choose to give your time to rather than mindlessly giving your precious attention to pointless things that drain your mental energy. Mindfulness is about observing the world in a nonjudgmental manner. Nonjudgmental doesn't mean you don't experience emotions while practicing mindfulness. Emotions aren't counterproductive to mindfulness. In fact, they are an integral part of the process. However, the key here is to know be able to let go these emotions effortlessly.

Here are some powerful ways to practice mindfulness in everyday life to fill the gap between your conscious and subconscious mind so that you can challenge negative notions held within the subconscious and transform them into more positive and productive thoughts.

Be Mindful of Where You Focus Your Thoughts

Leave rumination to the cows, not your thoughts! Do not allow unproductive and pointless thoughts to occupy your mind for long. Be intentional about the kind of thoughts that you allow in your mind. Think of the space in your mind as premium real estate. Only the very exclusive elite can rent space here. Only thoughts you choose to give your energy to can make their way into your mind. You get to pick what type of people can reside rent space here.

The type of thoughts that make their way into your mind is determined by you alone and nobody else. You have complete power and control over your thoughts. Make an effort to purposefully focus on things rather than letting the mind wander. If the mind wanders for a bit, gently acknowledge these thoughts and try and draw attention to the thing that you choose to focus on.

For instance, let us say you decide to practice being more mindful in your daily life. You take a train to and from work every day. During the journey, instead of thinking about what you'll cook for supper or how you'll convince a potential client to sign up for a deal, try to be in the present. Observe the beauty along the route to work. Watch out for the trees and flowers. Be more mindful of the people around you. How does it feel to sit in the comfortable seat? Practice thinking only about the things and people who want to think about or focus on.

Control your realm of focus. Be more mindful of where the mind wanders when it does. Bring your attention slowly to the present if you find yourself thinking about the past or worrying about the future. Before controlling focus related to what is happening inside you, try to control focus on external factors. Focus only on what you choose to focus on.

Increase awareness of actions

Mindfulness is a type of awareness but it isn't the same thing. Practice greater awareness in your daily actions in an intentional manner. Look at the motives behind your actions rather than simply being aware of your actions. What is the intention and purpose of the action? A majority of people go about their life in a mechanical manner, acting and responding to things as required. Often, there is no thought behind our responses and actions. Paying attention to the tiniest details while acting or reacting will help a person take stock of their thoughts and how they want to be driven by these thoughts.

Lend Purpose to Actions

Focusing on your actions is a part of giving your acts a greater sense of purposefulness. The purpose can be choosing to give something your attention or being completely present as you go about accomplishing tasks. Be aware of who you truly are, what thoughts you hold in your mind, and the purpose behind your actions and responses.

Ask yourself the purpose behind doing something for every action. Make your existence more purposeful and intentional. Focus all attention on what you are experiencing in the present moment and the feelings it is bringing within you.

Avoid Living in The Past or Future

Don't dwell on the past or be anxious about the future if you want to practice greater mindfulness. People have the tendency to ruminate about past actions and be hung up on feelings of guilt and regret. Thinking excessively about the past is not compatible with mindfulness. The past cannot be changed, no matter what you do. The present moment is what you have to make the necessary changes in your life.

Each time you find your thoughts wandering into the past, purposefully drive them back into the present. Absorb lessons from past events without focusing too much on them or without letting them affect your present.

Again, avoid being anxious about the future. There's nothing wrong with making plans for the future, however, don't be consumed by them. When these future plans impact your daily life, and you lose sight of the present, the purpose of mindfulness is defeated. Mindfulness is all about focusing your attention on the present moment and experiencing it to its fullest. When you are thinking about a grocery list while eating your lunch, you aren't practicing mindful eating. Instead of living in the now, you are worrying about the future.

While planning for the future is great, don't be so taken over by the idea that you lose a grip on the present. Worry and anxiety about the future are in opposition to the core principles of mindfulness. Don't speculate or think too much about the future at the cost of appreciating what is presently occurring in your life.

Avoid Looking at the Time

I know most of us are slaves of time and work to the command of clocks. We keep looking at the time every now and then to check how long it has been since we began an activity or when we need to start the next activity. Stop living your life like a machine based on the dictates of time and start concentrating on the present moment.

Of course, looking at the time per se is not a problem. However, don't focus too much on the passage of time if you want to be more mindful. Practice going through the day without looking at the clock frequently. Don't fuss about how long you have been waiting for something or someone.

Instead, start appreciating what is happening in the present moment.

Allow Yourself Do Nothing Sometimes

Multitasking and being productive is fussed about a lot in the current world. I am not advocating being unproductive all the time. However, at times it is alright to do nothing. It is alright to spend time alone, to calm the mind in a quiet environment and focus on witnessing the world around you. This is also a form of meditation. Sitting peacefully to empty the mind and focus on experiencing the present in its purest form.

Release Negative Emotions and Be Non-Judgmental About Thoughts

When you are more focused on the present, you will end up noticing a bunch of things you may not have been aware of before. Through observation, these things become more noticeable than before. A vital aspect of mindfulness involves being more mindful or aware of what is going on around you without assigning judgment to it.

Try to be more objective while noticing your surroundings. Avoid the urge to blame, judge or look down on others.

Instead, be compassionate and empathize with them. Similarly, resist the temptation to judge your own thoughts when you closely observe them.

By staying in the now, it is easier for you to adapt a nonjudgmental approach towards others. Our judgment often arises from the point of determining how our or someone's actions impact the future. When we stop living in the future, the tendency to judge other people and our own thoughts reduces.

Avoid Holding on to Emotions

Clinging to emotions is the opposite of mindfulness. Being mindful is about mastering the ability to let go of what has happened in the past and the emotions attached to it. When you truly live in the present, you learn to appreciate positive moments rather than worrying about their end. Avoid worrying about the fact that these moments will end in the future and appreciate their existence in your life at the moment. Similarly, resist the urge to compare present moments with moments that preceded them in the past. Whether your past moments were as eventful or your future will be as interesting is not important. Don't lose the present in your quest for comparisons with the past and future.

Trust Your Inner Feelings

Mindfulness involves living in the present and releasing judgments, worries, and regrets. It doesn't advocate being stoic or emotionless. Rather, you should acknowledge and embrace emotions. However, simply let these emotions pass once you acknowledge them rather than letting them take over your life. Think of these emotions as weather that eventually passes without you having much control over it.

Negative emotions are similar to thunderstorms that descend upon you without prior warning. However, thinking excessively about a thunderstorm doesn't make it disappear sooner. Allow positive and negative emotions to come and go. Let them go. Avoid clinging to them to the point that your mind is overcome by past regret or future anxiety.

Chapter Seven: Guided Visualization

Guided Visualization and Imagining Your Future

Don't you sometimes believe that you are almost operating on auto-pilot? We go about our lives in rush mode, often not stopping to think about why we do what we do. There seems to be a clear, well-defined method through which we operate without questioning it. Our commitments to our family, community, and society are so overwhelming that we often feel stressed under the weight of it. To quieten the conscious mind and tune in to higher levels of consciousness we need to be in a more relaxed state.

Guided meditation can be used to accomplish personal goals, change the pattern of your thoughts, still the mind and gain a deeper awareness of the self. An athlete can enhance his or her performance by visualizing their performance on the field. Similarly, a person who is afraid of public speaking can visualize him or herself confidently addressing an interested and inspired bunch of people. Visualization often helps you accomplish personal goals because they are detailed and function at a deeper level.

It can also be used to deepen your awareness of yourself. If you want to tap into your subconscious mind to comprehend why you feel the way you do, guided visualizations may help you uncover the truth. Through specific thoughts, ideas and images, you may be able to unlock answers to questions that were previously baffling. Sometimes, you'll struggle to find answers to certain questions through your conscious mind.

For example, you may struggle to determine which career option is most suitable for you and practice guided visualization to gain a sort of awakening or insight based on the knowledge held within the subconscious and unconscious mind.

Visualizing Future Through Guided Meditation

Here's how you can practice guided meditation to visualize your future.

You can record verbiage for this on audio or video and play it each time you want to practice visualizing your future. Play a soothing, serene and relaxing piece of music in the background.

Choose A Peaceful and Relaxed Place That Is Free from Distractions.

Sit straight/upright on a chair. Shut your eyes. Take a deep breath and completely relax your senses. Don't fall asleep, just go into a deep state of relaxation and keep your mind open to imagination.

Think about your present life. Think about everything that is important to you in your present life. Visualize your family and friends. Think about where you are professionally. Visualize working in your office or workplace.

How do you feel when you visualize the current happenings in your life? Take some time to reflect on how you feel about your current life.

Think about a goal that you desire to accomplish within a year from now. Do you want to be in a more meaningful and fulfilling relationship? Do you want to get your degree? Do you want to take a break and travel? Do you want to quit your present job and helm a start-up? Do you want to get a promotion? Think about a single goal and dwell on why it is so important to you to manifest it. How will accomplishing this goal add value to your existence? In what way will it make your life better? Think about all these things. Visualize the goal continuously within the mind's eye.

Relax completely and try to penetrate into different layers of consciousness by being aware of all thoughts related to your goal. What are the thoughts, ideas, images, and feelings you get when you think about the goal? How do your body and mind feel when you visualize the goal?

Go one week into your future. Where do you see yourself one week from now where your goal is concerned? If you want to go to university, have you filled the acceptance or admission form? If you are nervous about addressing an audience, have you signed up for a public speaking class or started practicing in front of a mirror?

If you want a dream job, have you identified it and applied for your dream job? What steps have you taken towards the fulfillment of your goal? What decisions have you made towards the fulfillment of your goal? How do you feel about embarking on the path to success or goal fulfillment? Imagine moving towards your goal slowly. Visualize eliminating all obstacles along the way.

Similarly, visualize yourself 2 weeks, and later six months into the future. What are the changes that have occurred in your life? Are you any closer to your goal? What are the emotions that occupy your mind as you inch closer to your goal? You are going forward continuously and are on the path to success.

Go further into the guided visualization session by looking one year into the future. Now, visualize yourself having successfully accomplished the goal. The success that you dreamt of is finally yours! Visualize yourself being successful in accomplishing the desired goal. What do you look like after having accomplished the goal? What is everyone saying to you? Who are the people you are mingling with? What are the typical things you do throughout the day? What are you saying to other people? How do you feel about accomplishing the goal? How does it feel to be successful? How do you sit, stand and walk? What clothes are you wearing? What are typical words you use? What do your surroundings look like?

Now rewind a bit and reflect on the entire process of accomplishing your goal. Visualize all the hard work, dedication and effort. How did you do to accomplish your goal in a step-by-step manner? What were the tiny changes you made to your life to achieve your goal?

What are the big changes you made in fulfilling your goal? What did you do on a daily basis to accomplish the success you are currently witnessing? What are the changes you made in your professional life? What are the changes you made where relationships are concerned? Did you make any internal changes for accomplishing success? Did you challenge certain pre-held notions, ideas, beliefs, and thoughts to achieve success? Take a moment to reflect on all the big and small steps you took to accomplish your goal.

Chapter Eight: Transforming Negative Thoughts Through Meditation

"It takes but one positive thought when given a chance to survive and thrive to overpower an entire army of negative thoughts." – Robert. H. Schuller

Negative thoughts are similar to wild beasts. However, the good news is like all beasts, they can be tamed. Even if you have acquired a series of negative, self-limiting beliefs about yourself over a period of time, they can be challenged. By working with your breath and focusing on your thoughts, meditation lets you treat each thought as a message that helps you receive signals from the mind. However, the best part is, the thought also carries information about how you can respond to the message.

For example, you may think you are not good enough, or you are helpless. This can be a signal from the mind that you need to reflect on what you should do to feel good about yourself.

Whenever you find yourself thinking you are not worthy of love, halt in your tracks. Slow down and show loving-kindness to yourself. When you tune into the real message behind these thoughts, the negativity starts fading. For example, in the above scenario, if you feel you are not worthy of love, the mind is signaling you to do things that make you feel more worthy of being loved.

Embrace Opposite Thoughts Meditation

Keep your eyes closed and sit in a comfortable position. Allow your mind to experience the sights and sounds around you. Notice the sensation of air against your skin. Notice the rhythm of your breath. Notice thoughts that occupy your mind and the sensations they trigger in the body.

Take a negative thought that has consumed your life lately. Do you think you are not good enough? Or you are powerless? Or completely shattered or broken? Do you regret not doing something in a particular way?

Notice the sensations in your body when this negative thought occupies your mind. Where do you notice a clear or focused sensation? Does it affect your heart, gut, stomach, throat and other areas of the body? How do you feel? Stressed, anxious and closed?

Now once you notice how this thought feels, challenge it! Think the exact opposite of the negative thought to condition your mind into greater positivity. Embrace opposite thoughts. So I am broken, and powerless is replaced with *"I am completely okay the way I am"* or *"I could've done this differently"* becomes *"I am always doing my best"* or *"I feel broken"* is replaced with *"I am complete."*

Affirm the opposite of your negative thought. How does your body feel? How do you feel in the heart, stomach, throat, and gut? Do you feel less tensed and more open? Notice the changes in your body.

Take time to explore each negative thought and turn it on its head. All along the session, observe the impact the two thoughts have on your mind and body.

Embrace Positivity Through Loving-Kindness Meditation

Start with yourself. Calm the mind, body, and heart, and define the center of your being or existence. Feel warm, compassionate, gentle and loving feelings towards yourself.

Loving-kindness or *metta* meditation is showing yourself and everyone around you inclusive and unconditional love. When you hold plenty of negative thoughts about yourself and others, loving-kindness meditation can help you gain more acceptance of yourself and others around you.

Keep a comfortable and relaxed posture. Focus on the heart center as you inhale and exhale from the heart center region. Imagine it to be the center of everything that is happening in your life. Notice negativity in the form of judgment, self-loathing, hatred and more. Go back to the strength and security of the heart. Continue breathing in and breathing out.

Move to a person who stands for unconditional love, a form of love that doesn't ask for anything in return. It can be a parent or a mentor or anyone who represents unconditional love for you. Show them love, respect, and gratitude. Visualize the person and show them unconditional love originating from the heart's center. Affirm your love for him/her by saying something like, "may she/he be blessed, safe, happy and protected all the time."

Next, move to a person who is neutral. Someone who you don't have a strong love or hate for. You neither like nor dislike this person. Feel a sort of tenderness, compassion and loving care towards the person. Wish them well and pray for their welfare. Similarly, show them love by saying, "may he/she be blessed, safe, happy and protected all the time."

Finally, move to a person you have hostile feelings towards. Someone who evokes feelings of hatred and resentment. This may be a person who has wronged you at some point in life and instilled negative feelings in you. It may be challenging to wish this person well. Say something like, "to the best I can, may he/she be blessed, safe, happy and protected." If you feel pangs of hatred for the person, move back to the person you love.

Let the heart experience feelings of loving-kindness once again before moving back to the person you dislike. Keep moving back and forth until you feel loving-kindness for the person despite a history of negativity related to him/her.

Bring about a shift in your subconscious mind about feelings related to the person.

Allow your words to pass through the entire body, heart, mind, and spirit. Strengthen your imagination to touch all beings in the universe with loving-kindness. Exist with all living beings until you feel a sense of unison and a serene profoundness or interconnectedness of all beings.

Expand the loving-kindness until you can visualize the entire planet spinning into the universe with a loving, kind energy. Keep expanding the realm of your positive feelings to make them as inclusive as possible.

Conclusion

Thank you again for downloading this book.

I sincerely hope this book was able to give you comprehensive, actionable straightforward and proven meditation techniques for fulfilling your personal goals and challenge self-limiting beliefs held in the subconscious mind.

The next step is to act by following all the simple yet highly effective meditation guidelines, consciousness tapping methods, and strategies to unlock the limitless potential of your subconscious mind. Identify a practice that works for you, and that you can connect with at a deeper level or combine a variety of techniques to establish a connection between the conscious and subconscious mind.

Begin today, for a person who reads without implementing valuable tips is no better than a person who cannot read. Knowledge is pointless if not applied in transforming our lives. Stop dreaming and start doing.

Lastly, if you enjoyed reading the book, please take the time to share your thoughts by posting a review. It'd be highly appreciated!

Visit my facebook page:

https://www.facebook.com/AlexChandLee/

Meditation: How-to

A Four Week-Plan to Deep Meditation

Table of Contents

Meditation How-to:

Table of Contents

Introduction

Chapter 1: Getting Back to Basics

Why should we learn to meditate?
I'm ready to start meditating, how do I begin?
Learning to meditate and relax is good for you
What can I expect from this 4-week plan?

Chapter 2: Establishing Your Practice

Why should I establish a meditation practice?
How I start a meditation practice?
Does what time of day you choose to meditate matter?
When I'm meditating, is there a specific posture I need to follow?
Making use of meditation anchors

Chapter 3: Week 1 - Challenges You May Experience

Common challenges faced during the meditation process

Challenge 1: I can't stop my mind from thinking, help!
Challenge 2: Sitting like this is making me restless
Challenge 3: Meditating is making me feel sleepy
Challenge 4: I'm so busy every day, how do I find the time to meditate
on top of everything else?
Challenge 5: My body aches sitting in one spot

Chapter 4: Week 2 - Fundamentals of Successful Meditation

Essential practices that help you meditate successfully
How to build a habit of regularly practicing meditation
How to discipline yourself and spend at least 30 minutes a day meditating

Pick a consistent time

Chapter 5: Week 3 — Traditional Meditation Postures and Exercises You Can Do

Variations of the sitting down position

The Lotus position
The Quarter Lotus position
The Burmese position
The Chair position
The Seiza position

Practical exercises for every posture to get your body ready for meditation

Neck rolls
Shoulder rolls
Stretching out the spine
Side bends
Leg bends

Chapter 6: Week 4 — Mindfulness Exercises to Get You Started

Mindfulness exercises you can try today to help you improve your meditation sessions

Exercise 1 – Mindful breathing
Exercise 2 – Awareness

Exercise 3 – Mental focus

Chapter 7: Deep Meditation in 30-Days

Achieve deeper meditation in 30-days
Day 1-5
Day 6-15
Day 16-25
Day 26-30
Thoughts to remember

Chapter 8: Tips to Get the Most Out of Your Meditation Sessions

Secrets & tips to experience deeper meditation

☐ Your intention for each session
☐ Calm yourself before starting
☐ Think happy thoughts
☐ Sit in silence before you begin
☐ Write down your thoughts
☐ Do yoga stretches
☐ Listening to music
☐ Meditating at the right time
☐ Getting the lighting just right

Conclusion
Description

Introduction

Congratulations on downloading this eBook and thank you for doing so.

If you're reading this book, you probably already have a good idea about what meditation is. You may be just starting out on your meditational journey, or you may already have been practicing this exercise for some time now, and you're planning to take your meditation sessions to the next level by achieving a deeper state of meditation. Either way, this book is an excellent guide to take on your journey as it will help you get the most out of your meditation sessions.

Ultimately, this book aims to prepare you for a state of deep meditation with a program that has been laid out to guide you towards achieving that goal within four weeks. Deep meditation is a quest that a lot of meditators seek to accomplish, but it is a process which takes time, and before you can reach that state of being, you need to get the basics done right.

In this book, you will discover how to improve your experiences with meditation. Whether you're a beginner or someone who has already been practicing this regularly, you will discover the fundamentals of establishing a successful meditation session, along with the challenges you may experience on your journey and how you can overcome them. You will learn helpful mindfulness exercises to help you get started before finally starting out on the four-week plan program to achieve that ultimate goal of experiencing a deep meditation.

The popularity of meditation is increasing, there is no denying that. After all, when you've discovered something that could benefit your life in such a tremendous way, wouldn't you be eager to start adopting it in your daily life? It is so much more than just a way to reduce stress and improve your happiness, meditation can help you build an increased sense of awareness, enhance your concentration, develop self-discipline and more which you will go on to read about in this book.

There are plenty of books on this subject on the market, so thanks again for choosing this one! Every effort was made to ensure it is full of as much useful information as possible, please enjoy!

Chapter 1: Getting Back to Basics

Meditation, it exists for a reason.

It's not just about reducing stress or letting go and taking a few moments to ourselves to try and recompose and regain our thoughts. Meditation is more than just that.

It is about finding balance, inner peace, and calm in a world where it seems that almost every aspect of our lives triggers so much stress, worry, or anxiety. Our bodies and minds may be strong and tough, but there is only so much negativity that they can take before this starts to take its toll and affect our health, sometimes to a point where it could become unbearable.

If only there were a magic formula of some sort where we could keep out these negative feelings that are capable of causing such destruction within our minds and bodies, but there isn't. Which is why we need to turn to meditation as a way of managing our worries and anxieties, to find a way to find that balance within ourselves and recharge our energy.

The beauty of meditation is that it is simple yet powerful. Simple enough that anyone can learn how to do it effectively with the right tools, teachings, and techniques. Anyone can learn the art of meditation, and it isn't as difficult as you may imagine. Sure, you may have tried it a few times and found yourself struggling in the early stages to quiet your mind and achieve a focused, calm, and mindful state. That is perfectly normal, especially if you're a beginner just starting out on this journey.

Mastering the art of meditation, like everything else, takes patience, time, and practice. You're putting far too much pressure on yourself if you expect to get it right from the moment you sit cross-legged on your mat and shut your eyes hoping to achieve deep meditation right from the get-go. No, it takes time and practice, and you need to be patient with yourself. In this book, you will find a four-week plan that will help you achieve deep meditation, and the key to succeeding in this is to remember that you need to be patient. Practice makes perfect, which is why your goal of achieving deep meditation is spread out over four weeks, you need time to master each stage and phase of the process before moving onto the next. With repeated effort and your goal clearly in mind, you will see results at the end of the four weeks.

Why should we learn to meditate?

Is it just about calming our minds and finding inner peace? This is a part of it, that is why a lot of people find meditation to be a helpful practice. Those who avidly do this find that their mind is peaceful and free from worries and mental discomfort, making it easier for them to achieve happiness compared to those who do not practice meditation at all. If you've never tried it, you may scoff at the idea that sitting quietly in a corner for a few minutes every day will make a difference in your life, but you would be surprised.

Think about it. What is it that successful people and motivational speakers often say they do as part of their daily routine? That's right, they spend a few hours meditating in the morning. Clearly, it's working for them, isn't it? Because they can make it through the difficulties of life, even with the struggles that may come their way, with a positive attitude, and they don't let stress get the best of them.

Now, you don't necessarily have to practice meditation in the morning the way they do, you can meditate at whichever time works best for you. There is no hard and fast rule. You can even meditate more than once a day if you need to and if you find that it helps. You make your own rules according to what you're comfortable with.

By spending a few minutes each day training your mind and making meditation a part of your routine, you will discover that your mind will gradually find peace a lot easier and finding happiness is something that doesn't seem so elusive anymore. Even if you have certain challenges that you may be facing in your life. Even in the most difficult of circumstances, you will find that you will remain calm, steady, and still, have the energy to look at the bright side of life.

Learning to control our minds is one of the most difficult things we can do. It's easy to let our thoughts get the best of us, which is why it is so easy to be consumed by the negativity if the seemingly hopeless situations we find ourselves in. The thing about this is, we don't even realize just how severely we are affected by it all because we're not really thinking too much about it. Fluctuations in our mood seem like a normal, everyday occurrence and we brush it off as being part of life because we can't control it. But that's where you are wrong.

Because you can control it with meditation. Create that inner space and clarity in your mind that will give you firm control over your thoughts, despite the circumstances you may be facing. Meditation is how you find that mental balance, so you're never at one extreme or the other (never too sad or never too happy). It's always about finding the right balance. You've always been told you need to live a balanced life and eat balanced meals. So why not have a balanced mind too?

Meditation is a way of bringing your mental clarity, and to change the way you look at the world around you.

At its very core, meditation is about taming your mind. A lot of people struggle with trying to overcome anxiety, despair, agitation, and other habitual thought patterns which they may find difficult to break out of. Taming the mind through mindful meditation is how you give yourself control of your own well-being once more. Meditation will bring you a sense of fullness and completion, and believe it or not, it is the only way to truly achieve tranquillity that is easily accessible to everyone on this planet. True, there may be other temporary forms of serenity, but nothing will come close to bringing you the long-term peace that you seek no matter what you may be going through in your life the way meditation will. And that is why we should learn how to meditate.

Meditation has been practiced traditionally for hundreds — if not thousands — of years, it is not something that just came about overnight as a new trend. Meditation is something that is inherent in all human beings, something we all have in us, something that we can all do. Many are already reaping the benefits of what meditation has to offer, and now it's time for you to start doing the same thing.

I'm ready to start meditating, how do I begin?

There's more to meditation than merely sitting cross-legged on your mat with your eyes closed as you breathe in and out, which you will understand as you progress throughout the rest of this book. There are many, many ways to meditate, but every meditation practice must begin with these most basic steps:

1. Know your intention

You must first set your intention before you begin your meditation. You need to have a purpose in mind, to remind you of why you are doing this in the first place. This intention is something you need to think about before you begin each of your meditation sessions. An example of this is that you hope to be less stressed, you hope you gain better mental clarity, you hope to learn how to balance some intense emotions that are going on in your mind right now, or you simply want to take this time for yourself to quiet your mind after a long and stressful day (if you're meditating at the end of the day). Meditation is all about being mindful, so make sure to think about what your intention is before each session.

2. Posture matters

In meditation, your posture is important. You need to breathe deeply and bring your attention inwards. You will be doing a lot of deep breathing during these meditation sessions, and you need to ensure your posture is right, or you're going to find yourself struggling to get through a lot of the pain and discomfort you might experience during the early stages of practice.

3. You must relax

The reason why meditation focuses on deep breathing is that you need to let your body relax. Mindfully focus on relaxing every muscle of your body during your meditation session, from your face, neck, and hands all the way down to your stomach area and other parts of your body. Being able to relax is key during a meditation session because you won't be able to quiet your mind if your body is a tense ball of anxiety. Whenever you may find yourself tensing up, you need to remind yourself to relax, relax, and relax.

4. Find your focus

If you're struggling to steady your thoughts during your meditation, it helps to have something for your mind to focus on. The easiest thing to do is to focus on your breath, to concentrate on breathing in and out slowly, rhythmically and methodically. Just focus on the in and out of your breath. During this time, you may find your mind wandering occasionally to other thoughts, and that's okay. Whenever you catch yourself being distracted, just slowly bring your thoughts back to your breathing once more. You'll get the hang of it soon enough.

Learning to meditate and relax is good for you

Meditation is good for your mind, body, and soul. It is so important for everyone to make time for taking care of their bodies, not just physically but mentally and spiritually too. Often we're just focused on taking care of the physical part of ourselves that we neglect to remember our minds need just as much attention and care because we don't realize the extent of what being weighed down by stress, worry, and anxiety can do to us. These negative emotions are so powerful that in some cases, they can severely affect our health.

We need to take care of our minds, and meditation is the way to do that. Among the benefits you stand to gain from consistently practicing meditation include:

- Reduction in your stress levels

- Improvement in your concentration and focus

- It improves your cognitive and creative thinking skills

- With greater mental clarity, you can make better decisions and solve problems

- An increase in self-awareness

- An increase in happiness

- An increase in self-acceptance because meditation helps you reconnect with your inner self

- It will help you learn to appreciate life more as you become more aware of your surroundings through mindfulness

- You learn how to block out distractions in your life

- It improves your breathing and your heart rate

- Helps you feel more connected to yourself

- It helps regulate your mood and anxiety disorders

- Helps you sleep better at night

- Helps lower your blood pressure levels

- Increases serotonin production which will help improve your mood

- You gain clarity and peace of mind

- Your problems seem more manageable when you don't let your mind get the best of you

- Increases your sense of well-being

- Helps you regain emotional steadiness

- It improves your mental resilience against adversity and pain

- It increases your optimism

What can I expect from this 4-week plan?

The following chapters will take a deeper look at what you can expect to experience during this 4-week journey towards achieving your goal of deep meditation. Each chapter will help you gradually build up towards your goal by exploring what you can expect to face and provide you with the tools and the exercises you need to overcome each obstacle you may meet during the process. By the end of each chapter, you will be better prepared, mentally and physically for what's to come. Be ready to dive into the 4-week program to successfully achieve deep meditation within 30-days with ease.

Chapter 2: Establishing Your Practice

As part of the four-week program to achieve deep meditation, you need to begin by establishing a practice for yourself first. Meditation may seem like an easy enough exercise, but it is an exercise that requires you to be mindful of everything that you're doing throughout the session. Meditation has a purpose and a goal, it teaches you to act with consciousness and to be mindful of everything that you do.

Why should I establish a meditation practice?

Just like a home needs a solid foundation on which the house can stand upon, so too does your meditation sessions. That foundation is developing a meditation practice of your own. Without a firm foundation to stand on, it won't be long before whatever you're doing eventually crumbles and falls because nothing is supporting it. That's just one way of describing how important it is to develop a sound meditation practice right from the very beginning of the process.

Although meditation is something that is beneficial for everyone, not everyone is currently putting it into practice. Some people are not practicing meditation at all. Why? Because it isn't a habit. That, and many of us lead very busy lives, sometimes our plates seem too full to take on anything else. There is always a reason not to start something, which is why it is entirely up to you to make time for it.

The purpose of establishing a meditation practice is that you want to make meditation a habit, a part of your daily life, something you're willing to do every day without even thinking twice or resisting it because you're hard pressed for time. Establishing a practice will make meditation an ingrained activity in your life, much like how brushing your teeth or showering, preparing something to eat, and even your daily commute to work. Those habits are so deeply ingrained in you that you can do them without any effort, nor do you put a lot of thought put into it.

That's what establishing a meditation practice aims to do for you right now, and something you need to establish as a foundation which will eventually lead to your four-week program to achieve deep meditation.

How I start a meditation practice?

The following steps will help you start establishing a meditation practice for yourself, preparing you to be well and truly ready for the four-week plan to achieve a deeper state of meditation:

☐ **Baby steps at first**

Trying to do too much too soon is how a lot of people crash and burn. You need to start small, and this can't be emphasized enough. Yes, it seems like slow progress in the beginning, but that's okay. Remember that old saying, "Slow and steady wins the race?" Keep the bigger picture in mind and practice patience. Start small at first by meditating for short periods of time, maybe 5-10 minutes a day especially if you're new at it. You can do anything for 5-10 minutes a day with no trouble, and the time will pass before you even know it. Once you see how easy it is, it keeps you motivated to keep challenging what you can do. Creating small, achievable goals you can do every day is how you begin building the habit of making meditation a part of your daily life.

☐ **Make use of apps**

Smartphones are another thing that has become so ingrained in our lives, many of us wouldn't know how to survive a day without our smartphones. There is an app for just about everything these days, even meditation, so why not make the most of the tools you have to help you establish a successful daily practice? There are several apps available that could help you enhance your meditation sessions, with everything from timers to ambient sounds to help set the mood. If it helps make your daily practice more enjoyable, why not? You're more likely to stick to something if you like what you're doing.

☐ Use guided meditations

There are apps that will guide you through the meditation process, and if you need to rely on one, in the beginning, go ahead and do it. Guided meditations can be a great tool, especially for beginners on this journey, to help you stay on track and on the right path. It will help you make sure that your breathing techniques are actually effective, that you're relaxed, it helps you visualize, and it helps you free your mind to immerse yourself better in the whole experience if you're not constantly focused on whether or not you're doing it right. Guided meditations make it much easier, especially for beginners to start getting into the flow of things and helps you progress in the right direction with your meditation sessions, even if you're doing it solo. It helps to know that you're heading in the right direction.

☐ Create your space

Creating a space within your home that you actually look forward to spending some your time in is an essential part of establishing a consistent meditation practice. Create a space in your home that is dedicated solely for your meditation sessions, and fill that space with anything you need to make you feel comfortable, that makes you feel like you want to be there for a while. You can fill it with pillows, cushions, pictures that inspire you, incense or scented candles if it helps, anything that helps soothe your soul and brings you a sense of calm. This will go a long way towards helping you make meditation a routine in your daily life. Having a space in your home that you look forward to spending some time in each day because of the comfort and calm that it envelopes you in can really help.

☐ Put it on your calendar

If you're just starting out, you need to have reminders so you won't forget to practice your meditation for today. Make it a point to mark it on your calendar or make a note of it using the calendar app on your phone. It can be easy for your other daily tasks to take precedence over your meditation session, which is why you need to purposely make that time to just stop and meditate before the day comes to an end and you realize you didn't get to spend any time meditating at all.

Does what time of day you choose to meditate matter?

As long as it works for you, you can choose to meditate in the morning, afternoon, evening, or even before you go to bed. That's the beauty of this practice, you have the freedom to choose whatever's comfortable for you. Every individual is different, and no one does things the exact same way other people do and have the same experience. Some people prefer to meditate in the morning because it sets the tone for the rest of the day, while some prefer to do it at night because it helps them unwind, calm down and relax after a really long and hectic day.

The best time of the day for you to meditate is any time that you can consistently and realistically commit to each day. It can be in the morning, in the afternoon, in the evening, at night, it doesn't really matter. As long as you're getting it done, that's the only thing that matters, even if it is for just 10 minutes a day. A short meditation session is better than not doing it at all.

When I'm meditating, is there a specific posture I need to follow?

No, there isn't because once again, everyone is different and some people may prefer one posture while someone else may prefer another. That's okay, the posture you decide to pick should be the one that you're most comfortable with and makes you happy. If sitting in a chair works better for you, go ahead and do that. If you prefer to sit cross-legged on a mat, that's alright. If you prefer to lie down, that's alright too. It is important to do what is right for your body and to do what you connected with the most as this will make you relax yet alert at the same time during your session.

Making use of meditation anchors

Even the most advanced meditation practitioners could use an anchor every now and then. Our mind is such a versatile thing that sometimes it can get easily distracted and wander before we become aware and bring it back to focus again. Which is why meditation anchors are helpful, especially if you're new to this practice, as they will help you find the focus and concentration you need during your meditational session. Even if you're an advanced practitioner, having an anchor will still help you whenever you have days where your mind is struggling to grasp the concentration that it needs.

A meditation anchor will allow you to steady your mind and maintain focus on what you are doing. An anchor gives you a point to bring your mind back whenever it deigns to wander off. An anchor gives you something to connect your mind as you strengthen and build your mindfulness, a practice you will eventually master in time.

A meditation anchor can be anything that you find useful, that helps you to maintain your focus. Some suggestions of what could be used as an anchor when you meditate include:

- ☐ Focusing on your breath as it moves in and out of your body

- ☐ What your body feels like with each deep breath you take

- ☐ Your chest as it rises and falls slowly and rhythmically with each breath that moves in and out

- ☐ If you're using music or any ambient tones to help set the mood, you can focus on that and the way it makes you feel as you listen to the rhythm

☐ Physical sensations that slowly emerge as you progress throughout the meditation, for example, the way your hands feel, or the way the muscles in your body feel

Are you starting to get the picture? Your anchor can be anything that you want it to be, it doesn't have to be restricted to a list. It just has to be something that you can connect on, something that your mind can focus on while you meditate. It helps you give a purpose, especially when you're just starting out. Otherwise, you could find yourself aimlessly sitting on a mat wondering if you're doing it right or if you're not doing it right at all.

This would be a good time to find an anchor that works best for you and can help you with your meditation practice. Bringing your thoughts back to your anchor whenever you need to is a great help in your four-week plan to achieve a deeper state of meditation.

Having a regular anchor is still helpful, but if you ever feel that you want to choose or use something else as your anchor, go ahead and do it. If it helps you stay focused and it works for you, your anchor can be anything you want it to be. Remember, it is all about finding what works best for you because meditation is an enriching experience, one that is entirely yours.

Chapter 3: Week 1 - Challenges You May Experience

As much as we would like things to be smooth-sailing all the time, challenges are an inevitable part of life. Then again, without challenges, it wouldn't be life, would it? If everything went our way all the time, how would we know when we improved or achieved something great?

While meditating, you're bound to run into a few challenges along the way too, especially if you are new to this practice. Even those who have been meditating for some time can find themselves up against an obstacle or two. It is important to acknowledge these challenges and accept that they are part of the journey to successful meditation. Often, beginners to the practice might give up completely if they find themselves struggling because they don't realize that it is perfectly normal to struggle in the beginning.

Meditation may seem like a simple, passive exercise, but don't be fooled by its simplicity. It can prove to be a challenge in its own way because this exercise isn't just about training your mind to calm your thoughts, but it is also actively training your mind to improve resilience, concentration, and mindfulness at the same time.

Let's take a look at some of the common problems and obstacles you're likely to encounter during your meditation:

Common challenges faced during the meditation process

Newbies and regular practitioners alike are bound to run into a challenge or two at some point during their meditation process. Here are some of the common challenges you can expect to face:

Challenge 1: I can't stop my mind from thinking, help!

It can't be emphasized enough how common this obstacle is. It is very natural to experience this, especially for beginners who have never attempted to meditate before. Getting lost in your thoughts is something that everyone does, it's just that you've never paid much mind to it, and when you're now actively trying *not* to think too much, that's when it seems like your brain is working overtime to think even more.

Here's how you can overcome this challenge:

- Use your anchor to help center your attention and reign in your focus. That's what anchors are there for, to help give you something to focus on other than your thoughts which are running around all over the place.

☐ Before you start meditating, say to yourself, "Stop!" and then immediately start to take a few deep breaths in and out so you can focus your attention on what you're doing.

• If you find your thoughts wandering away from your anchor, that's okay. You don't have to get too stressed about it, just stop yourself once more and actively go back to concentrating on your anchor. Your mind will eventually calm down, don't worry.

Challenge 2: Sitting like this is making me restless

This is not uncommon. Some people may find it hard to sit in one spot for too long a time, especially if they were already agitated or anxious before they began. Or maybe you've just had a really stressful day, and all that pent-up energy is still running high, and you're finding it difficult to sit still and quiet your thoughts. You're trying, but you still feel restless, and it's disrupting your mind, preventing you from successfully meditating. It can be difficult for the mind to relax when it's in a state of restlessness.

Here's how you can overcome this challenge:

1. First, don't be too hard on yourself because you're not doing anything wrong in this scenario. What you need to do is mindfully acknowledge that yes, you are restless and it's affecting your concentration. The mind has a tendency to get caught up in its own world, and that is perfectly normal.

2. Rely on your anchor again to help you get settled down, and if you need to, turn to external sources to help induce feelings of calm. For example, listening to music until your mind feels relaxed enough to begin the meditation process.

3. If you need to, go for a short walk to release some of that energy, and then come back again and try to meditate once you feel that you've calmed down immensely.

4. Concentrate and turn your thoughts towards your body, noticing the areas where you feel most tense, and then try to make a conscious effort to relax those muscles. Take deep breaths, keep repeating to yourself, "Relax"

and focus on how your body feels, whether the tension is leaving your muscles and if you slowly start to feel yourself unwinding. As you slowly begin to relax, you'll find yourself calming down, and the restlessness begins to leave your body.

If you need to, switch positions or find a different spot to meditate in if that helps. You could even try walking meditation, which is where you walk at a steady pace but incorporate all the meditation practices such as focusing on your breathing. Begin by walking at a moderate pace as you try to release some of that restless energy, and then gradually slow down your pace. Remember to keep concentrating on breathing in and out.

Challenge 3: Meditating is making me feel sleepy

Another common challenge. This tends to happen when your body is too relaxed and not alert enough to what you are doing so the mind triggers you to think that you're feeling sleepy. Which is why it is important to remain alert and mindful during your meditational sessions, and you can do this by having something to focus on.

To overcome this, here's what you need to do if you find yourself getting sleepy during your meditations:

- Sit up straighter, open your eyes for a minute and refocus your attention on what you're supposed to be doing.

- Rely on your anchor once more to help center your thoughts and to keep you alert during the session.

Challenge 4: I'm so busy every day, how do I find the time to meditate on top of everything else?

This is completely understandable. We lead hectic and busy lives, where we always seem to be on the go from the moment we wake up in the morning and right to the time we're ready for bed. Every task you have on your plate is going to seem important, things that need to get done, that it doesn't make sense or feel right for you to spend some time meditating when you could be getting things done. There is always a reason not to do something, and things always seem to come up. How are you supposed to find the time to meditate on top of everything else you've got going on in your life?

Here's what you can do:

- Yes, you are busy, and there's so much going on, but one thing that can help is to remind yourself that you need to take care of yourself first. If you don't look after your health, both mentally and physically, you won't get anything done since you let yourself become sick.

- It is helpful to remember that meditation helps keep your mind, body, and soul in optimum condition, which will benefit you even more in the end because you can get more done if you're at your peak condition. Spending 15-30 minutes a day is a small time-out for yourself which you need — and more importantly, you owe it to yourself — to do because you only have one body and one mind, and it is your responsibility to take care of it the best you can.

Challenge 5: My body aches sitting in one spot

That's bound to happen especially in the beginning because you've never done this before. Your body is bound to experience some discomfort during this new experience, muscle cramps, and aches being the most common. It can be hard to concentrate when your body is feeling discomfort.

Here's what you can do:

☐ First, if you're feeling uncomfortable, you want to check if you're sitting properly and your posture is what it should be. Bad posture is something we don't pay much attention to because we don't even notice it. We could be walking around with bad posture all day and not even realize it. An obvious sign that shows you if you have bad posture is that you will feel uncomfortable pretty quickly, so try readjusting your position and your posture.

☐ Switch postures if sitting cross-legged on the floor is something you find too uncomfortable. This cross-legged position is known as the 'Full Lotus' position, and it can be quite demanding especially for beginners. So it's alright if you need to try something else instead. Try sitting on a chair if it helps, or lie down if your back is hurting too much every time you try to square your shoulders and not slouch.

☐ Try doing some simple stretches before you commence your meditational session to loosen your muscles and help your body relax a little. Sitting in one spot when you're feeling tense and strained can make it even harder for you to get comfortable.

Discomfort and challenges are all part of the process. You're doing something that your body probably isn't used to doing, so don't get discouraged if you're struggling to get it right in the beginning. It's okay to take a break from your session and come back to it again when you feel ready, you don't have to force yourself to struggle through the process. Meditation is supposed to be a relaxing and calming exercise, and there's no point trying to finish a session if you feel no different from when you started.

Chapter 4: Week 2 - Fundamentals of Successful Meditation

It seems like there's a lot to take in, isn't there? It can be overwhelming at first when you find out that meditation isn't simply about positioning yourself comfortably on your mat with your eyes closed, and that there's a lot more that goes into the process than you may have initially realized.

Everyone who tries their hand at meditation wants to do it successfully the moment they start. Now, while meditation is a very personal thing and an entirely unique experience for different people, there are still some fundamentals which you can rely on to help you achieve a successful meditational session.

Essential practices that help you meditate successfully

These practices are not too complicated, nor are they too restrictive, that's the good news. You might be surprised to find just how simple the fundamental secrets to successfully meditate are. If you're ready to begin your journey to achieve a successful meditation, here are five fundamental steps you can keep in mind to achieve optimum success during your sessions

- **Don't have any expectations**

Yes, you probably had expectations before you started this practice and you didn't even realize it. But pause for a moment and give it some thought. Did you decide to begin meditation expecting to get something specific out of each session? If you did, you need to learn how to let that go. Meditation sessions are different, some days will be easier than others while some days will seem longer than others. If you go into it with expectations in mind, you're only setting yourself up for disappointment if things don't go your way. So, let go of any expectations and approach each session with an open mind and the possibility that anything can happen. Whatever comes, just go with the flow and meet it without resistance.

- **Choose your right fit**

Remember how there is more than one way to meditate? This is great because it gives you the option of finding what works best for you. Explore the different methods of meditation until you find one that you love the best, it will make it easier to have successful sessions that way.

- **Create the perfect environment**

Your environment matters, and if you've ever tried meditating in a space that wasn't conducive to meditation, you will see that there's a very big difference indeed. Your environment should not only be one that is set-up to infuse you with feelings of calm and relaxation, a space that you look forward to spending time in, but it must also be a space that is quiet, free of noise, clutter, bright lights, devices and anything else which could prove to be a distraction. Your environment should promote a feeling of peace and serenity, somewhere you can't wait to rush home to and spend some time in, that way you will look forward to each session and immerse yourself completely in an enriching experience.

* **Be mindful throughout the day**

One of the purposes that meditation plays is to bring a greater state of mindfulness, teaching you to pay more attention to your surroundings and be conscious of your actions and your feelings. Being in a state of mindfulness doesn't have to stop the minute your timer goes off to signal meditation time is over. Instead, exercise mindfulness every moment you're awake and as you go about your daily routine. No matter what task you may be handling at the moment, do it with mindfulness and focus. In other words, give each task your complete attention. This will help you sharpen your focus, and you will see what a difference this makes when you undergo your meditation sessions.

How to build a habit of regularly practicing meditation

Before you can reach the deep meditation that this book will help you accomplish with the 4-week plan program, you need to practice meditation on a regular basis. Think of it as swimming, you don't just jump into the deep end and expect to be a fantastic swimmer that knows all the right strokes from the minute you hit the water. You need to start at the beginning and work your way up to the deeper end of the pool.

Meditation works the same way. You need to regularly practice meditation before you can accomplish a state of deep meditation, which is taking it to the next level. The best way to do that is to make it a habit of practicing meditation every day if possible, but at least several times in a week. Meditation needs to be a part of your life the way eating a meal is. It has to be something that you want to do every day without fail.

How to discipline yourself and spend at least 30 minutes a day meditating

You can start small of course, but at least 30-minutes a day is what you eventually want to work your way up to because that's a part of the 4-week plan program. The best way to start disciplining yourself to do this is simple, you need to reflect on why this is important to you. Why did you decide to take up meditating in the first place? What did you hope to accomplish through this practice?

Finding out why is how you find the drive to keep going and to stick to what you set out to do. Without a reason, you're going to flounder and eventually give up altogether, because nothing is pushing you to keep going. Remind yourself why you decided to make a commitment to do this, write it down on a post-it note and stick it all over your house and workspace if it helps remind you to keep going. If you've been struggling to develop the habit, try the following methods to help you along the way.

- **Start small, with just about 2 minutes**

Thirty minutes is what you want to eventually achieve. If you're just starting out, don't sweat it, just start small and work your way up from there. Starting with 2-minutes each day is more than good enough to get the ball rolling, and once it becomes a habit, it'll be easier for you to go for long periods without even noticing it.

- ## Work with others

Joining a friend or a group of people who have the same goal as you do can go a long way in helping you build a habit of making this a regular practice. Knowing that you're not alone on this journey can prove to be a tremendous form of support. Doing so also establishes a sense of belonging. Plus, having the company makes the activity more enjoyable, especially if you're the sociable type who likes being around others often.

- ## Remember you're doing this for yourself

When was the last time you did anything for yourself? When have ever taken the time off to focus on you and what you need? We get so busy and caught up with everything going on in our lives it's easy to let our own needs slide or just be completely forgotten altogether. But you owe it to your body to make sure that you take care of yourself. You're doing this for yourself, and no one else. You're doing this so you can reap all the benefits meditation has to offer you, and no one else. You owe it to yourself to step back from everything that is consuming you each day and spend sufficient time recuperating and recharging yourself.

- **Let go of your judgments**

If you're going to constantly berate yourself whenever you think you're not performing as you should, meditation won't be a very pleasant experience for you, nor will it be beneficial in any way. Meditation is about letting go of the things that hold you down emotionally and mentally, and this includes letting go of your need to be perfect all the time. Don't be too hard on yourself whenever you stumble along the way, it's how you learn to get better and become better. Instead of fixating on how you think your meditation session should go, just let go and immerse yourself in the experience, no matter what may unfold in your life.

Pick a consistent time

Understandably, your schedule is likely to be different each day. To develop a habit where you never forget to meditate, try and assess your regular pattern throughout the week. Compare that record a couple of weeks later and see if there are any drastic changes or movements in your schedule times. And from there, pick a time of day which you think would work best every day of the week and every week. It doesn't have to be a specific time per se, just a general one like deciding you will meditate in the morning before breakfast, in the afternoon, during your lunch hour, or even at the end of the day before you go to bed. Sticking to a regular time frame each day will help you develop the habit much easier.

Chapter 5: Week 3 — Traditional Meditation

Postures and Exercises You Can Do

Have you ever sat down during a meditation session, especially when you first started, and wondered if you were doing it right? Especially when there's a lot of different postures and positions you could do. Before you embark on the 4-week deep meditation program, you'll need to get the postures and positions perfected.

There may be a lot of different postures and positions, but you will find that a lot of people who are meditating will often look quite similar. There are some elements of meditation where the postures are universal because it is the best way to calm the mind and connect and align your body for maximum effect.

Let's explore these meditation postures and exercises which you could practice until you get them right, so you're ready to handle what comes in the 4-week deep meditation program up ahead. Let's begin by looking at the different types of traditional meditation postures, followed by the types of practical exercises you can do to get your body ready for these poses.

Sitting down on the floor or on a mat in a cross-legged position is one of the most common pictures that spring to mind when someone mentions the word 'meditation.' If you've never done this before, be warned that this position can get quite uncomfortable after a while because you're not accustomed to sitting down for a long period of time with your legs crossed. Feeling tingly or aches in your legs after a while, or even aches in your back are normal especially if your posture isn't quite right.

Variations of the sitting down position

There are several ways to position yourself on the floor, and sitting cross-legged is just one of them.

The Lotus position

The first variation is called the 'Full Lotus,' which is the posture most commonly associated with meditation. Here, you would need to sit with your legs crossed, and both your feet resting on the opposite thigh. Your index finger and thumb are touching each other, and you will rest these on your thighs, palms facing upwards, sitting with your back straight. This is the ultimate yoga pose and requires that your hips be open throughout the practice. To avoid experiencing any muscle aches, do some light stretches to loosen up your muscles before commencing this position. If you're dealing with muscular pain and backaches, try leaning back against a wall for added support. If it helps, it is fine to use a cushion to sit on to make yourself more comfortable. Stretch out one leg at a time, and slowly bend it in towards the position before doing the other leg. Take your time getting comfortable.

The Quarter Lotus position

The second variation is called the 'Quarter Lotus' position. Like the Full Lotus, except this time your legs can be loosely crossed in front of you without having to be placed on top of your thighs. In this position, you can have both feet resting below the opposite knee, and if you find the Full Lotus too uncomfortable, you can opt for this version of the position instead. Your hands can be similar to the Full Lotus, with your thumb and index finger touching, palms facing upward and placed over your thighs, or you can have your palms pressed together in front of your chest, elbows facing out. Again, you need to do some light stretching first before commencing this position, stretching out your legs and your back especially. It is completely fine to use a cushion if you need to sit more comfortably, and it is alright to lean against a wall to support your back.

The Burmese position

The third variation is called the 'Burmese' position. In this position, you would sit with your back straight, but your legs do not have to be crossed the way they are like the Lotus positions. If you're having difficulty getting comfortable with the Lotus, then this position would be ideal for you. Sit with your back straight, with both your feet lying on the floor in a more relaxed position. Your feet would look like the Lotus, but instead of placing one on top of the other, this time both feet are on the floor next to each other (still cross-legged). Beginners find this method the most helpful to start with before they progress further and start practicing the Lotus position. Just like the other positions above, stretch out your leg muscles and your back especially before commencing the posture.

The Chair position

If sitting on the floor is too difficult for you, you can sit down and meditate in a chair instead. Starting out in a chair is sometimes one of the best ways for beginners to get used to the practice of meditation. If your body is having trouble sitting on the floor, sitting on a chair is perfectly fine too. Sitting on a chair also helps with maintaining a straight spine throughout the position instead of leaning against a wall. Be sure to use a straight-backed chair for this practice, and sit with your feet firmly touching the floor. You should be sitting forwards in your chair, not relying on the back of the chair to fully support your spine. Your goal in this position is to sit relaxed, yet upright so that you can still maintain alertness.

The Seiza position

This is another variation of the 'sitting down' position, except instead of sitting with your legs crossed on the floor, you will be kneeling instead, using a cushion or a rolled-up mat placed between your legs for support. You will be kneeling forward, with your feet tucked underneath your buttocks, and the cushion or rolled mat place between the back of your thighs and near your feet.

Practical exercises for every posture to get your body ready for meditation

To really immerse yourself deep in your meditation, you need to be comfortable. You will find it hard to concentrate on achieving a calm and peaceful state of mind when you're distracted by the aches and pains happening in your body after a while. You could ignore it for a while, but the longer you progress, the more it will get to you until you're eventually restless and just waiting for the session to be over, which defeats the purpose of meditation, to begin with.

Here are some practical exercises you can do before every meditation posture that will help your body loosen up, relax, and sit comfortably for much longer. You want to do these exercises, especially during the four-week program because achieving deep meditation will require you to sit for at least 30-minutes or more.

Neck rolls

This exercise will help you loosen your neck muscles and release all the tension and stress you may be carrying at the back of your neck. Start by loosely dropping your chin down to your chest, remember not to tense anything. Once in that position, slowly and gently roll your head from one side to the other. First, roll it to the left, hold it there for a couple of seconds, and then roll it to the right. Do this a couple of times until your neck feels nice and loose. Then move on by rolling your head up, tilting your chin towards the ceiling, hold it there for a moment, and then roll it back down again.

Shoulder rolls

This is a really good one to follow those neck rolls because our shoulders are where we next carry our tension and stress. Now that you've loosened up your neck, you need to work on doing the same for your shoulders. You can either sit or stand when you do this, whatever works best for you and then roll your shoulders slowly. First roll them forward for a few seconds, and then roll them back for a few seconds, and repeat as many times as necessary until you feel nice and relaxed. When you're done, just allow your shoulders to fall into the relaxed position and keep it there for a moment while you enjoy that feeling.

Stretching out the spine

Backaches have become a norm for many, especially those who spend long hours sitting behind a desk at work. It is important to stretch out your spine because if you're suffering from backaches, you're going to have a difficult time getting through the meditational postures, a lot of which require you to keep your posture nice, strong, and straight. Start in a standing position, bringing your feet close together. Place your palms together in front of you, and slowly lift your arms above your head, keeping your palms together the whole time. Lift it up as high as you can, while keeping both feet firmly on the ground. Imagine there's a hook at the top of your head that is pulling you upwards to really get into the stretch as much as possible so you can stretch your spine all the way. Hold for a couple of seconds, relax and bring your palms down towards your chest again, and repeat the motion.

Side bends

It is important to stretch out the sides of your body as well as the spine, and that's where these side bend exercises come in. Start in a standing position with your feet slightly apart. Inhale and stretch one arm over your head, then slowly bend towards the opposite side, keeping that arm above your head and bending over your head as the other arm rests by the side of your leg. Just like stretching out your spine, you want to imagine there is a hook pulling you as far towards the side of your body will allow you to go. Hold it there for a couple of seconds, really getting into the stretch, release and do the same thing on the other side.

Leg bends

Stand with your feet slightly apart, and place your hands on your hips. Slowly lift one leg, with your knee bent as high as you can go. Hold it there for a few seconds while keeping your balance, lower your leg back down and repeat the same thing with the other leg. After you've gotten comfortable doing this a few times, take it a step further by extending your leg out slowly when you lift it, holding it for a few seconds before bringing it back down. This helps to stretch out your hamstring muscles even more.

Chapter 6: Week 4 — Mindfulness Exercises to Get

You Started

We all want to enjoy the bountiful benefits which deep meditation brings. Even regular meditation is beneficial, and that's why many start out on this journey to begin with. With a goal to improve their mind, body, and soul.

We live in a busy world that is constantly tugging at our focus and our mind, pulling it in several different directions every day that it is easy to lose yourself and your focus along the way. Achieving overall wellbeing and happiness means taking care of your mind just as much as you take care of yourself physically.

Meditation is a tool which we can use to cultivate a positive mind and a balanced body. As we explored earlier, in week 2 of the plan, you may find it a challenge to reign in your thoughts and maintain your focus during your meditational sessions.

Now that you've covered the essentials, weeks 1-3 will prepare you for the deeper meditation session. Week 4's mindfulness exercises are the final step you need to get you well and truly ready. We've covered the challenges, the fundamentals you need as the foundation for your success and exercises to help improve your posture, which is the physical part of meditation, and we're now ready to move onto preparing you mentally for the deep meditation process.

Mindfulness exercises you can try today to help improve your meditation sessions

Mindfulness is just as important for a successful meditation session as maintaining good posture and position is. These mindfulness exercises will help you sharpen your focus, which is one of the most crucial factors for a successful meditation session. Without mastering the skill to focus, you're going to find it a constant challenge to keep your thoughts under control and to immerse yourself in your meditative experience. The best part is, you only need 3 exercises to help you improve your meditative experience!

These 3 exercises are easy to follow, and they can be slotted into your daily schedule whenever you have a free moment. If you have the time to spare, you can even spend a few extra minutes on these mindfulness exercises before beginning your meditation sessions. If you don't, that's okay too, you can easily perform these exercises at any time throughout the day when your time permits you to.

Exercise 1 – Mindful breathing

Breathing is an essential part of the meditative experience, so it is only natural that we should exercise this too. Whenever you meditate, you're breathing mindfully as you focus on each purposeful breath that goes in and out of your body. Mindful breathing doesn't just have to happen when you're meditating, it can be done anywhere and at any time whether you're sitting, standing or just walking about. Make it a habit to breathe mindfully, and you'll find it much easier to do so during your meditation sessions.

1. Start by bringing your attention and focus on your breathing.

2. Breathe in slowly for approximately 3 seconds, and then release that breathe slowly, counting to 3 seconds again.

3. During this exercise, you should focus and think of nothing else except your breathing. Do not think about the tasks you need to do, like a meeting that is coming up at work. Think about nothing except your breathing in and out, counting the seconds as you do.

4. Concentrate on the air that is filling your lungs as you breathe in, the way it makes your body feel, and when you release your breath, imagine all the stress and the tension leaving your body as you do.

You can do this for 1-2 minutes at a time throughout the day, several times a day and you're already on your way towards improving each meditation session when you get better at learning to control your breathing.

Exercise 2 – Awareness

When you meditate, you learn to become more aware of your body, your mind, and your thoughts, aware of what is happening all around you when your eyes are closed because your other senses become heightened when your eyes are shut. Being mindfully aware helps you sharpen your focus and remain alert not just to your surroundings, but to your thoughts as well. For example, if you are mindfully aware of your thoughts, you will have better control when it comes to keeping any negative thought or emotion at bay.

Exercising your awareness throughout the day will help sharpen your alertness towards everything around you. Not just around you, but within you too. Beginners often find focusing on awareness to be a struggle in the beginning, because it's so easy to let our thoughts drift and get distracted by everything else. Training yourself to be more aware will help you connect your mind and body better during your meditation sessions. So it's a good idea to practice these throughout the day to help you sharpen your focus and cultivate a heightened sense of awareness.

1. Start by choosing an activity or an object to focus on. Pick something that you would normally do without thinking twice about it, like opening the door or getting dressed in the morning for example.

2. Once you've got your object or activity, start to really, actively pay attention to what you're doing. If you're opening the door, concentrate on it. Reach for the doorknob and be aware of how it feels in your hand, and the motion of pulling the door towards you or away from you. Stop and appreciate how lucky you are to be healthy and fit enough to walk out your front door with a destination and a purpose in mind.

3. When you're getting dressed in the morning, focus and be aware of what you're doing instead of just going

through the motions. Concentrate on how the fabric of your clothes feel in your hand, and even stop to appreciate how fortunate you are to have a selection of clothes to choose from as you go through your closet looking for something to wear.

4. Before you eat, be aware of the food that is in front of you, how good it smells, the shapes, the colors. As you take each bite and begin to chew, be aware of how the food tastes and you take each bite with purpose.

Eventually, being mindfully aware is something that will come much easier, and the more you practice, the easier you will find it is to concentrate on what you're doing or thinking without becoming easily distracted by other thoughts around you.

Exercise 3 – Mental focus

Successful meditation involves being able to concentrate and not letting your thoughts to spiral out of your control, which means you need to work on improving your focus. Exercises to improve your focus are simple enough, here's what you can do:

1. Pick an object to focus on and place it in front of you.

2. When you're ready, set a timer and keep your focus on the object and nothing else.

3. Concentrate on that object and keep staring at it for as long as you can.

4. When your mind begins to wander, stop and make a note of how long you managed to concentrate on that object before your mind started to drift.

5. Next round, do the same thing but try to go for a longer time this time around, aiming to beat your previous record.

Gradually, you will be able to focus on the object in front of you for longer periods of time before you find yourself getting distracted. The longer you can focus on the object, the better your focusing abilities will become.

Chapter 7: Deep Meditation in 30-Days

Right now, you've already been equipped with everything that you need to unlock the power of your mind and attain a new sense of calm. Life doesn't have to be a big ball of stress when you know how to achieve a deep, meditative state. You now have an understanding of the meditation basics, the challenges you'll likely encounter, the different kinds of posture and the exercises to prepare your body, along with the mental exercises you need to help sharpen your focus for this deep meditative process to be a success.

Achieve deeper meditation in 30-days

Before you begin, there are a couple of things which you need to prepare yourself for to attain a deeper state of meditation. First, it is important to ensure that you are 'clean,' both on the inside and out. The outside is pretty simple, and everyone keeps themselves clean anyway. Having a nice, hot shower before your session will help you feel refreshed and energized, which is always a great feeling to start a meditation session with. But what is more important is keeping yourself clean on the inside too.

"Clean on the inside" here means not to consume anything before your meditation sessions that can alter your state of mind or make it difficult for you to concentrate. Avoid things like alcohol, coffee, medication and even avoid eating before your session. Having a full stomach or being intoxicated can make it difficult for you to concentrate when your body is busy digesting food or consuming any kind of substance that can alter your state of mind is just going to make it pointless to even try to meditate because you won't be able to focus enough to do what you need to do.

Ready? Let's begin.

Day 1-5

During the first five days of this process, you have to commit to spending a minimum of 30 minutes in a space that is quiet and comfortable. It is important that this space be quiet and free from any kind of distraction. Leave your mobile phone and other devices outside and forget about them for the next 30 minutes.

When you're ready, close your eyes and begin your mindful breathing. Concentrate on nothing except your breath for the next 30 minutes. By now, hopefully, you would have practiced your focus exercises which will help you do this for 30 minutes without becoming distracted. Even if you get momentarily distracted, your awareness by now should be at a point where you can immediately snap your thoughts back to where it should be.

This will be all that you need to do for the first five days of the process. By the end of the five days, you should be able to meditate with deep concentration for 30 minutes, and once you do, you can now move onto the next stage of the process.

Day 6-15

From day six to fifteen, you will now bring your body towards what is known as the 'hypnagogic state.' The hypnagogic state is a state of deep meditation state where your mind is somewhere in a transitional state from sleep to wakefulness. Where before you were alert and fully focused during your meditation, you will take it up a notch and free your mind even more.

Get settled in a comfortable position and empty your mind through your mindful breathing motions. Slowly begin to let yourself drift off almost like you would if you were sleeping. Allow your body to relax even more, while still being mindful of the way you feel throughout the process. Once you feel yourself dozing off (which happens when you're relaxed enough), pull yourself back to the hypnagogic state and remain there as long as possible. If you experience any visions, random thoughts, or hallucinations in the moments where you're about to doze off, don't worry, that is a completely normal part of the process.

By the end of day 15, you should be able to keep your mind suspended in the state between sleeping and dreaming while remaining in complete control. If it helps, you can play soothing music during the process to help you achieve a deeper state of relaxation.

Day 16-25

During these next few days, you're going to do something during your meditation sessions that you may have never done before, visualize. Create the perfect scenario in your mind, one that induces you with feelings of complete calm, peace, tranquility, and serenity. Hold that vision in your mind and picture it like you're really there and imagine as if it is right in front of you. If you imagine yourself meditating by the beach, create an image so real that you believe you are actually meditating by the beach. The visualized scenario can be anything that you want it to be, as long as it helps you achieve a state of deep relaxation.

And when you visualize, you're going to lose yourself completely into that image in your mind. Immerse yourself so completely and absolutely in that vision that you completely lose track of time. Be so immersed in your vision that you will lose all of your thoughts until they're completely gone from your mind. In this state, you no longer have to fight your thoughts and struggle to remain focused, you're already doing it. Remember to keep breathing deeply throughout this process.

Visualization is about decluttering your mind, and flushing out your thoughts so you can achieve a Zen state of mind.

Day 26-30

By this stage, you will notice a significant improvement compared to your previous meditation sessions before you embarked on this 30-day deep meditation plan. Your thoughts have achieved a state of stillness, and your body feels at peace, along with a sense of calm.

Your goal during the last few days will be to remain in this meditative state for as long as possible. It's easy to achieve this state, to maintain it and avoid outside distractions from destroying your focus is the real challenge. This is all you need to do during the final four days, you must gain the ability to maintain this state. Aim to do at least 30 minutes of it, but if you can go for longer, go ahead and do it.

As your deep meditative sessions come to an end, instead of opening your eyes hastily, exit from it slowly and gracefully, letting it happen naturally. Bring your mind back to the present and as you get ready to open your eyes and resume your normal routine once more, take a few deep, mindful breaths and slowly open your eyes. Your deep meditation session will leave you feeling energized and with a renewed sense of calm, happiness, peacefulness and gratefulness.

Thoughts to remember

Like everything else, meditation is an exercise and a process that takes practice and repetition to achieve the highest results. The more you practice, the better you will become, so don't get frustrated with yourself if the progress isn't what you expected it to be. Be patient and keep practicing, you will eventually get there in time.

Chapter 8: Tips to Get the Most Out of Your Meditation Sessions

As you can see, there's a lot more to meditation than meets the eye. It looks simple enough and sounds simple enough, but often many are surprised by just how much of a challenge meditation can prove to be. Anyone can still meditate of course, but achieving deep meditation is something that requires a lot of commitment, persistence, perseverance, and lots of practice. It may take you a while to get there, but the journey will be worth it when you start to experience how much of a difference meditation can make in your life.

Secrets & tips to experience deeper meditation

Achieving a state of deeper meditation is about proper technique and having the knowledge about what you need to do, but that's just one part of it. The other is knowing the secrets and helpful tips which will improve your meditation sessions even more so that deep meditation no longer becomes an elusive concept.

Want to experience deeper meditation? Follow the tips below so you can make the most out of your sessions:

> ## Your intention for each session

Having a purposeful intention for each of your meditation sessions is one way to do it. Make meditation a part of your everyday routine, but be careful because you could run into the risk of making it too routine, where after a while you're going through the motions like you would any other habit. That's not what we want to achieve. Enter each trance with pure intent, a desire to achieve something out of it and watch how your sessions transform completely just with this one simple change.

> ## Calm yourself before starting

A lot of people don't make the time to clear their thoughts or calm themselves down before beginning a meditation session. It's fine if you're doing your sessions in the morning after waking up because your mind is not yet boggled by everything that has gone on during the day. But if you're doing your sessions at the end of the day or in between, calming your mind is an essential tip that you need to make a part of your practice. Everything that we see, hear and experience throughout the day will have and leave an impact on us, whether we realize it or not, and if we attempt to enter a meditative state with our minds clouded by other thoughts, it's going to make it harder for you to concentrate. Make sure you take a few moments to walk around, relax, loosen up, and clear your head before you begin. You'll find it much easier to achieve a deeper meditative state that way.

> ### Think happy thoughts

This isn't just a saying that's reserved for the movies, it actually makes a difference in your meditation sessions. Meditation is about improving your happiness, and deeper meditation can help you achieve that. Before you do, however, you need to surround yourself with happy thoughts and expel any negativity that may be lingering on your mind. When your mind is in a state of joy and content, it is naturally more relaxed, and it quiets down a lot quicker than when it is plagued by worries. Thinking happy thoughts infuses you with feelings of appreciation, happiness, love, and joy, and going into a mediation session already feeling good about yourself will make it that much easier for you to concentrate. Thinking happy thoughts is easy, all you need to do is remember something that you are feeling grateful for, something or someone that makes you happy, or even the little things that happened during the day which made you smile and lifted your spirits.

➢ Sit in silence before you begin

If you're having a hard time getting into the relaxed state you need to be in before you begin your meditation, one thing that helps is sitting in silence for a few moments. Find a place that is absolutely quiet, and just sit in silence, that's all you need to do. Sit in silence and wait until your mind settles down on its own. When you're sitting in silence, it makes it easier for your mind to slow down and start to calm itself. This complements your meditation session because it will allow you to achieve a deeper meditative state since your mind is not buzzing with other distractions.

➢ Write down your thoughts

Another great way to quiet the mind is to give your thoughts an alternative escape outlet. Instead of having them compiled and jumbled together in your mind with no place to go, write them down instead. You can either write them down on a piece of paper which you can later throw away, or if you like to journal, you can keep a thought journal and write down everything you're feeling there. Pouring out your feelings and putting them down on paper is essentially giving your thoughts an escape outlet. If you've ever done this exercise before, you will notice how much better you feel after you've poured it all out. It's like talking to someone, except this time you're free to say absolutely anything without holding back because no one will know about it except you. Doing this before a meditation session can do wonders to free your mind.

➢ Do yoga stretches

Our bodies get stiff and sore from moving around all day, even more so if we sit behind a desk for several hours working away in an office. When your body is still, and your muscles are tense and sore, it can be difficult to achieve a deeper meditative state which requires you to be completely relaxed in both mind and body. Regularly doing yoga stretches will bring your muscles and your body some much-needed relief, and you will notice the difference when you meditate.

➢ Listening to music

Music is a very powerful tool. As the saying goes, "Music soothes the savage beast." Not that we are savage, but it gives you an idea of just what a powerful instrument music can be, and the profound effect it can have on people. Soothing music during a meditation session can do wonders to engulf you with a sense of calm and tranquility, and you will find it much easier to sink into a deeper meditative state with the help of the right kind of music.

➢ Meditating at the right time

You need to be in the right frame of mind if you're going to meditate. It's not just about sitting down on the mat, closing your eyes and waiting for the magic to happen. You may have the right posture and all the right tools you need, but if you don't have the right frame of mind, you're not going to achieve the deep meditation that you want. Avoid meditating when you're feeling bored, restless, lethargic, or disinterested because that's a sure-fire way to quickly lose interest, and you won't follow through with the session that you started. You won't be thinking clearly, and you'll subconsciously be resisting it because it's not where you want to be right now. If you're not in the right frame of mind, don't do it and wait until you're ready.

➢ Getting the lighting just right

Finding a quiet room is the first part of the recipe that you need for a successful deep meditation session. The second part of that is to ensure that the room has the right kind of lighting. Low lighting can relax the mind a lot quicker than fluorescent or bright lights will, so consider filling your room with natural or soft lighting. Candles work well in this instance.

Conclusion

Thank you for making it through to the end of this book, we hope it was informative and that it provided you with all of the tools you need to achieve your goals whatever they may be.

Meditation is a fantastic tool that can work wonders for your mind, body, and soul. You owe it to your entire being to take care of yourself in the best possible way and not just physically too. The body is a wonderful, miraculous machine, with so many aspects working in tandem with each other to help us live the best life we can. Meditation helps you look after yourself both on the inside and out.

You should be able to see the difference after your first deep meditation session, but if you don't get it right straight away, that's quite alright. Remember, one of the important key aspects to remember about meditation is to let go of your expectations and just go with the flow of things. Keep practicing it, and in no time at all, you will find yourself consistently achieving a state of deep meditation for longer periods instead of just 30-minutes at a time.

It brings you a world of benefits, everything from improving your concentration and increasing your happiness to reducing your stress, all aimed at encouraging you to live your life as the best version of yourself. People from all over the world have been reaping the benefits of meditation for thousands of years. You see successful people talking about it and touting meditation as a habit they make it a point to include as part of their daily ritual. Why? Because its effectiveness has been proven time and time again, and now you have everything that you need to do the same.

When you improve every aspect of your life, you will find that everything else falls into place. A life with less worries, anxieties, and stress, a life of enhanced relationships with the people around you, mental clarity to see the path in front of you that will lead you towards achieving every goal you have ever dreamed of and more. All of that is now yours for the taking, all with the simple yet effective practice of meditation.

Finally, if you found this book useful in any way, a review on Amazon is always appreciated!

Visit my Facebook page for free download and events

at:

https://www.facebook.com/AlexChandLee/

Description

Would you like to live a life where you are imbued with a true sense of fulfillment, happiness, peace, and serenity? Would you like to live a life where you will eventually feel happy and fulfilled, balanced even if you're in the most difficult circumstances or challenges that would otherwise have weighed you down mentally and emotionally?

A life like that is completely attainable, and it is among the many reasons why people all over the world have turned to meditation for the betterment of their health and wellbeing, mind, body and soul. Meditation is a way to calm the mind and attain a sense of inner peace, and it is the only effective long-term method that has proven to have real benefits which will free your mind from the worries, mental stress, anguish, and the challenges you have that your life may bring. The worries will be there of course, but the act of meditation gives you control over the way you feel instead of letting the emotions run your life.

Deep meditation is your key is gradually attaining peace and a purer form of happiness, and it is something that everyone can do. Everyone — yes, everyone — can learn the basics of meditation and eventually attain a state of deep meditation, unlike anything you have ever experienced before.

One thing's for sure, learning deep meditation is one of the best things you will ever do for yourself.

ALEX CHAND LEE

After a decade of stressful and hectic activity as professional stock trader, Alex overturned his lifestyle, returning to his ancient true passions: meditation, physical exercise and a simple and healthy lifestyle.

Hence the need to write, to direct those who have become overwhelmed by his same routine towards the rediscovery of a more "Humane" world, a world in which contact with nature and meditation become vital elements that draw the path to self-awareness and peace of mind.